MW00993207

VOLUME II

INTEGRATIVE MANUAL THERAPY

FOR THE UPPER AND LOWER EXTREMITIES

An Integrated Systems Approach Introducing

- Muscle Energy and 'Beyond' Technique for Peripheral Joints
- Synergic Pattern Release with Strain and Counterstrain
- Myofascial Release, A 3-Planar Fascial Fulcrum Approach

Sharon (Weiselfish) Giammatteo, Ph.D. P.T.
Edited by Thomas Giammatteo, D.C., P.T.

Revised Edition

North Atlantic Books
Berkeley, California

Integrative Manual Therapy for the Upper and Lower Extremities

Published by
North Atlantic Books
P.O. Box 12327
Berkeley, California 94712

Cover and book design by Andrea DuFlon
Revised edition by A/M Studios
Photography by John Giammatteo
Printed in the United States of America

Integrative Manual Therapy for the Upper and Lower Extremities is sponsored by the Society for the Study of Native Arts and Sciences, a nonprofit educational corporation whose goals are to develop an educational and crosscultural perspective linking various scientific, social, and artistic fields; to nurture a holistic view of arts, sciences, humanities, and healing; and to publish and distribute literature on the relationship of mind, body, and nature.

Library of Congress Cataloging-in-Publication Data

(Weiselfish) Giammatteo, Sharon
Integrative manual therapy for the upper and lower extremities / by Sharon (Weiselfish) Giammatteo, edited by Thomas Giammatteo
p. cm.
Previously published: Berkeley, Calif.: North Atlantic Books, 1998.
Includes bibliographical references and index.
ISBN 1-55643-260-7 (trade paper: alk. paper)
1. Extremities—Diseases—Treatment. 2. Manipulation (Therapeutics)
I. Giammatteo, Thomas. II. Title.

RC951.W448 2001
617.5'8062—dc21

00-054623

2 3 4 5 6 7 8 9 / 05 04 03 02 01

ACKNOWLEDGMENTS

I would like to take this opportunity to thank all those whose instruction, support and encouragement contributed to this book. My husband, Tom Giammatteo, D.C., P.T., contributed his time, effort and skill to make this book possible. Lawrence Jones, D.O., founder of Strain and Counterstrain Technique, was a significant influence. Frank Lowen contributed his perception and insight for the development of my "Listening" skills. All of my colleagues at Regional Physical Therapy in Connecticut participated in the implementation of single-subject design research to help refine the techniques in this book. Most of all, my clients were always ready to try anything new which might help.

Many thanks to John Giammatteo for his gift of photography, and to Ayelet Weiselfish and Genevieve Pennell for their contributions of art work.

My appreciation, once again, to Margaret Loomer, whose creativity and skill made this book a reality.

My sincere appreciation is extended to my best friend, Jay Kain, who has shared in my research and development of new material for many years.

Gratitude is extended to Richard Grossinger, publisher, and Andrea DuFlon, designer. My best efforts could not have produced this text without their intervention.

My love to my wonderful family, Tom, Nim, Ayelet, and Amir for their personal commitment to the success of this book.

Thank you.
Sharon (Weiselfish) Giammatteo

ABOUT CLINICAL RESEARCH AND THIS TEXT

I would love to describe in depth the clinical research which guided me to publish the contents of this book. Hundreds of patients have received all of the therapeutic interventions presented in this book. Thousands of clients have received some of the therapy outlined in this book, by myself, my associates, and other practitioners of manual therapy. The material in this text is almost all unique, the outcome and synthesis of my knowledge, skills, and "listening" abilities. Experience with all client populations, orthopedic, neurologic, chronic pain, pediatric and geriatric, has granted me an exceptional opportunity for learning.

Quantitative research studies have been performed on four hundred severely impaired joints with impartial "pre and post testing," using Myofascial Release, the 3-Planar Fascial Fulcrum approach. Otherwise, single subject designs are the common research approach incorporated into my clinical practice. I could have performed quantitative research studies for all of the unique techniques presented in this book, but then it would be several years before this text could be published. My preference was to publish this book, at this time; within it is important information for the health care consumer. I sincerely hope that practitioners will use this information with their clients to meet their individual needs.

Good luck and health.
Sharon (Weiselfish) Giammatteo, Ph.D., P.T., I.M.P.,C.

TABLE OF CONTENTS

FOREWORD

I have been fortunate and honored by a close working relationship with Sharon (Weiselfish) Giammatteo for many years. The effect she has had on my personal and professional growth has been one in which the status quo is rarely satisfactory and the words "can't" and "never" have been replaced by "anything is possible" and "always."

The first lecture I heard from Sharon in 1982 was truly representative of the passion she has for sincerity, integrity, and truth in a professional field where new information is often frowned on, ridiculed, and frequently vehemently opposed. While discussing a new concept of a systems approach for evaluation and treatment, she interjected a statement about the common overuse of ultrasound by many physical therapists. I was amazed to observe the majority of the audience either go completely silent or get extremely fidgety over the prospect that they were guilty of a common infraction. In other words, no one wanted to hear something that shook their reality. The paradigm shift was too great. With that statement and Sharon's thirst for continued practical knowledge, this scenario has been repeated more often than I can remember. Sharon's own learning encompasses a constant search for new and better ways to treat the whole person. Each bit of information she gains is immediately integrated into what she already knows, and quite often new and unique ways to treat people are created.

This Muscle Energy text is the direct result of that precise learning mode. While her first Muscle Energy text comprised remnants of her early learning from many of the field's top osteopaths, chiropractors, physical therapists and allopaths plus her own research, this new text encompasses totally new constructs taken as an application of the biomechanical principles she learned then and now newly applies. The product is a classic culmination of Sharon's learning and processing style in regard to applied biomechanics and a natural complement for her other integrative work. Sharon is the consummate student, researcher, and clinician when it comes to one of her greatest passions, biomechanics of the skeletal system. Not surprisingly, this work, already four to five years in process, has been refined to make its application simple, powerfully effective, and efficient and nonaggressive to both the patient and the therapist. When mastered along with the constructs in her first text, this book creates a solid cornerstone for the treatment of a majority of the body's biomechanical dysfunctions. Her newer research regarding cranial and transitional or Type III biomechanics sheds even further insight into the study of structure and function of the skeletal framework.

Sharon's research and clinical efforts have continued to cast light into unexplained and unexplored areas of applied biomechanics and clinical kinesiology. The work is grounded in core Newtonian-Cartesian physics but at the same time embraces the concepts of quantum physics and beyond.

Sharon's ability to facilitate and create new learning paradigms in different realms will most likely cause friction for those individuals who resist change or fear the unknown. Their facile reaction will be to deny the material, but their challenge will be to put as much energy into understanding and growing from the new knowledge as they would in opposing it.

I look forward not only to the dispersal of this material but the excitement and energy Sharon will put into her next text and the enthusiasm that she'll expend taking many of us on the journey to even greater health, harmony, and professional satisfaction.

Jay B. Kain, Ph.D., P.T., A.T.C., I.M.P.,C.

CHAPTER 1

POSTURAL COMPENSATIONS OF THE UPPER AND LOWER EXTREMITY JOINTS

The results of a comprehensive postural evaluation can facilitate a more effective and efficient treatment process. Posture is evaluated on a sagittal plane, a coronal plane, and a transverse plane. It is important to stand with a neutral base of support during all standing posture evaluations. The feet should be acetabular distance apart with approximately 15 to 20 degrees of equal external rotation of the feet. It is important to note that one foot is not slightly in front of the other. The knees should be equally flexed/extended. If there is recurvatum of one knee, it should be maintained in sagittal plane neutral to reflect similar posture to the other knee.

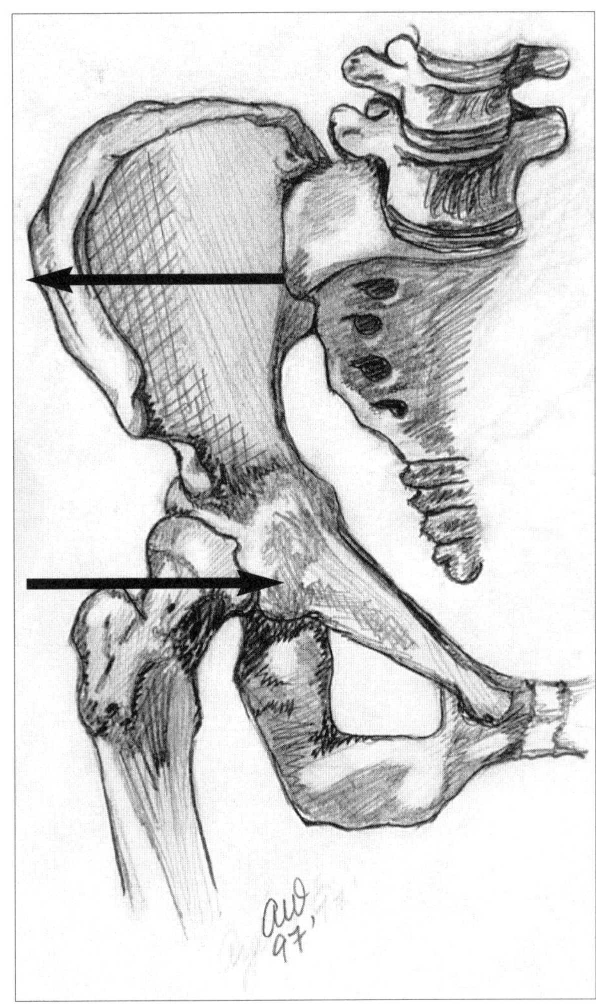

Figure 1. Typical Compensatory Postures: The pelvis will typically present a *lateral shear.* There is, typically, a decrease in the convex curve on palpation of the greater trochanter secondary to the compression of the femoral head.

Philosophy: Posture Reflects Movement Potential

Limitations of physiologic motion (flexion, extension, rotations and side bendings) should correlate with static posture evaluation. Postural deviations indicate the body's potential for dynamic movement. Consider whether there are mild, moderate, or severe neuromusculoskeletal dysfunctions.

Mild, Moderate, or Severe Postural Indications

- Severe dysfunction will cause severe limitations in ranges of motion with severe positional imbalance of the articular surfaces. Pain and compensation patterns will be observed in inner ranges of motion. Postural deviations will be considerable.
- Moderate dysfunction will cause moderate limitations in physiologic ranges of motion. Pain and compensation patterns will not be observed until mid-ranges of motion. Postural deviations will be moderate.

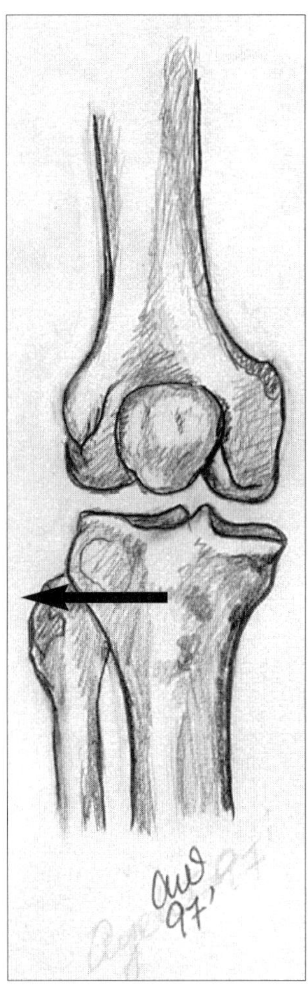

Figure 2. Typical Compensatory Postures: The proximal tibial articular surface will shear lateral.

- Mild dysfunction will only cause mild limitations in ranges of motion. Pain and compensation patterns will only be observed in outer ranges of motion. Postural deviations will be slight.

Assessment of Postural Dysfunction is performed to assess the body's capacity for normal joint mobility, soft tissue flexibility, and physiologic ranges of motion.

A Compensatory Pattern

Articular balance is the normal neutral relationship of two articular surfaces of a joint throughout a full physiologic movement. When there is joint and/or soft tissue dysfunction, the body will *compensate* in order to attain movement goals. Compensations typically occur at joint surfaces, and result in loss of articular balance.

Pelvic and Lower Extremity Posture

Observe in supine, prone, and standing. Observe postural deviations on three planes: sagittal, coronal and transverse. Observe articular balance of all joints. Document articular postural deviations of the knees, such as shears and rotations of the proximal tibial articular surface. Observe postural deviations of the feet: supination, pronation. Observe specific joint deviations of all ankle and foot joints (malleolus, navicular, cuboid, first ray, etc.)

Lower Extremities: Typical Compensatory Postures

- The pelvis will shear lateral (Figure 1).
- The femoral head will be approximated, caudal, adducted and internally rotated (Figure 1).
- The proximal tibial articular surface will shear lateral and externally rotate (Figure 2).
- The distal tibial articular surface will glide posterior (Figure 3).

- The talus will glide anterior (Figure 3).
- The distal fibula head will shift inferior and posterior (Figure 4).
- The calcaneus will invert (Figure 5).
- The foot will be pronated or supinated.

Neck and Upper Extremity Posture

Observe in supine, prone, sitting and standing. Observe postural deviations on three planes: sagittal, coronal and transverse. Observe articular balance at the joint surfaces. Document articular postural deviations of the neck, shoulder girdle, elbow, forearm, wrist, hand, thumb and fingers. Observe at the joint surfaces.

Upper Extremities: Typical Compensatory Postures

- The neck is side bent away from or towards the side of the shoulder girdle obliquity (elevated shoulder girdle).
- The head is rotated opposite the direction of neck side bending.
- There is an elevated shoulder girdle (shoulder girdle obliquity) (Figure 6).
- There is a protracted shoulder girdle (Figure 6).
- There is an abducted scapula (Figure 6).
- The humeral head is caudal, anterior and compressed in the glenoid fossa (Figure 6).
- The humerus is adducted, flexed and internally rotated (Figure 6).
- The elbow is flexed.
- The ulna is abducted (Figure 7).
- The proximal radius head is anterior (Figure 7).
- The distal ulna head is anterior.
- The distal radius head is posterior.
- The forearm is pronated.
- The proximal carpal row is anterior.
- The wrist is in anterior shear during extension.
- The thumb is flexed, internally rotated, and adducted.
- The proximal head of the first metacarpal is in anterior shear and compressed.

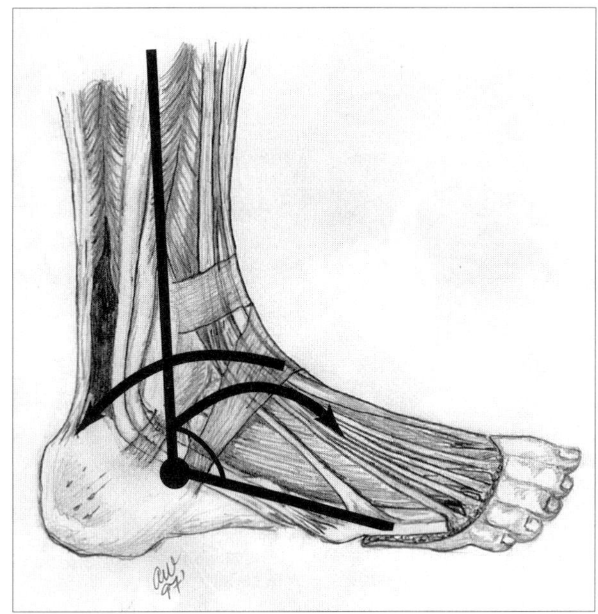

Figure 3. Typical Compensatory Postures: The distal tibia glides posterior, while talus glides anterior. The person is standing in plantar flexion (extended ankle). Extension forces will be transcribed up the leg during standing and ambulation.

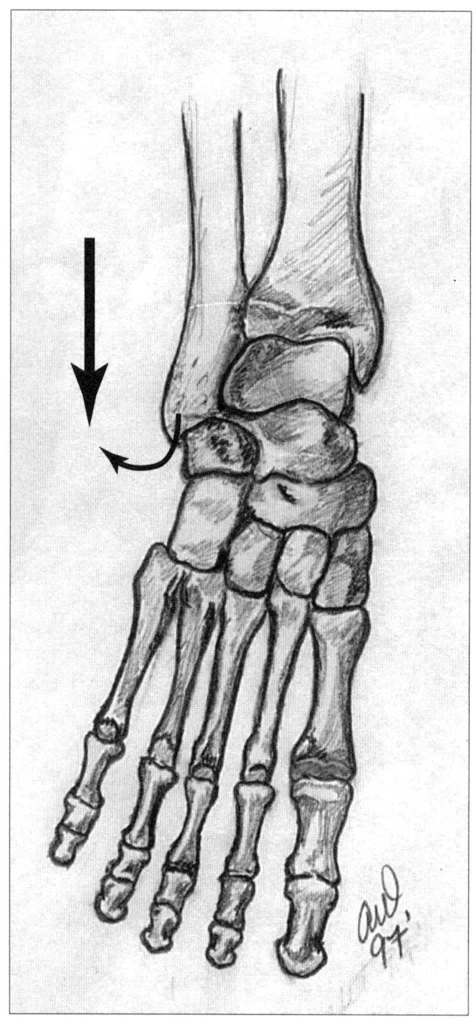

Figure 4. Typical Compensatory Postures: The distal fibula head is hypomobile, stuck inferior and posterior.

Movement Corresponds with Postural Deviations

Observe deviations during movement from midline neutral. Assess right-left symmetry, and limitations in ranges of motion. *Fixate* to inhibit compensatory *trick* movements, which occur because of poor articular balance. Limitations of ranges of motion should correspond with compensatory patterns observed during static postural assessment. For example, a protracted shoulder, observed in a static posture assessment, will present limitation in horizontal abduction during dynamic movement testing.

Articular Balance of all upper and lower extremity joints assures closed and open kinetic chain function.

Postural deviations *reflect and correlate with* articular imbalances, including in the hard and soft joints of the body. Examples of these joints are as follows:

- Soft tissue to soft tissue (e.g., liver to diaphragm)
- Soft tissue to bony structure (e.g., cecum to right ilium)
- Bony structure to bony structure (e.g., humeral head to glenoid fossa)

These joints *reflect and correlate with* compromised joint mobility and limitation of soft tissue elongation, which reflect and correlate with limitations in ranges of motion, which reflect and correlate with compromised function.

Hypomobility and Hypermobility

In the field of manual therapy, hypermobility is not typically an issue to be addressed. True hypermobility, with ligamentous laxity, in cases such as pregnancy and rheumatoid arthritis, are not the common causes of neuromusculoskeletal dysfunction treated with manual therapy. If there is a glenohumeral joint inferior dislocation or subluxation, this joint is not hypermobile in manual therapy concepts. The humeral head is hypermobile on one plane in one direction only: caudal. In all other planes (superior glide, posterior glide, etc.), and in all directions of physiologic movement (flexion, extension, abduction, adduction, and rotations) there is hypomobility. The humeral head is hypomobile. A dislocated glenohumeral joint is therefore a hypomobile problem. Manual therapy should address the neuromusculoskeletal dysfunction causing the hypomobility. The result of therapy for a caudal dislocation of the shoulder joint should be normal articular balance of the glenohumeral joint (i.e., a more normal superior position of the humeral head in the glenoid fossa.)

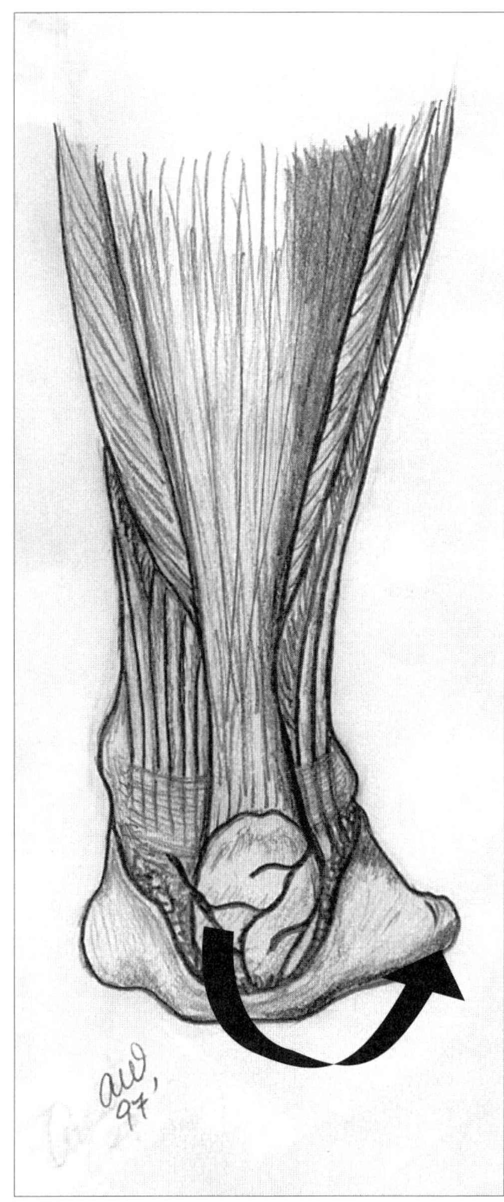

Figure 5. Typical Compensatory Postures: The calcaneus will invert.

Articular Balance and Accessory Movement

When there is a compromise of articular balance, with postural dysfunction, there will be a limitation in the accessory movements and the joint play of the joint surfaces. As an example, with a protracted shoulder girdle, there will be hypomobility on mobility testing of all joints which contribute to the shoulder girdle complex: costovertebral joints, costotransverse joints, sternochondral joints, costochondral joints, scapulothoracic joint, glenohumeral joint, acromioclavicular joint, and sternoclavicular joint.

Accessory Joint Movement and Physiologic Ranges of Motion

Whenever there is hypomobility of the accessory movements and joint plays of a joint, there must be correlating limitations in physiologic ranges of motion. There may be hypertonicity (protective muscle spasm) of the musculature surrounding that joint. There may also be fascial dysfunction of the connective tissue surrounding that joint. Yet if the body receives a command from the brain cortex to move the joint, the person will attempt to move and to reach the *movement goal,* in spite of the hypomobility. In order to attain the movement goal, the body will over-

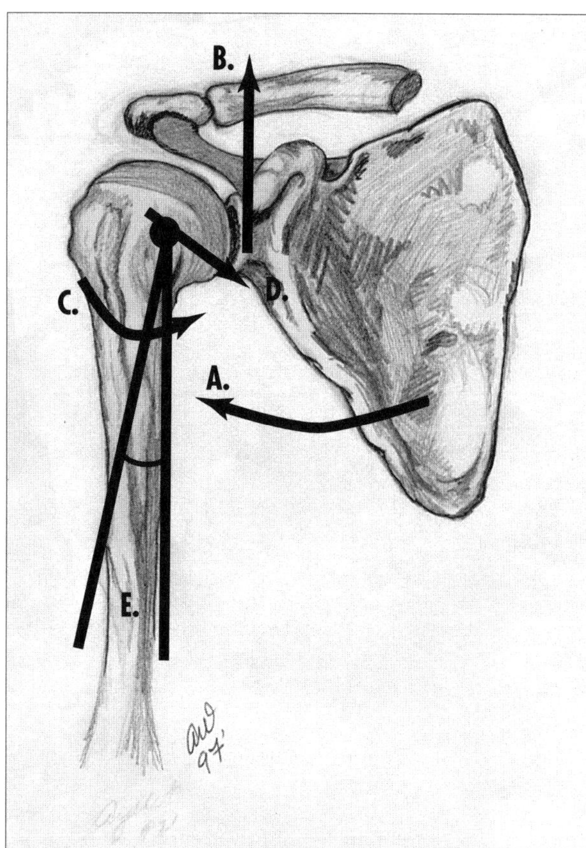

Figure 6. Typical Compensatory Postures: The shoulder girdle presents in this typical dysfunctional pattern: **A.** abducted scapula; **B.** elevated shoulder girdle; **C.** protracted shoulder girdle; **D.** anterior, caudal, compressed humeral head; **E.** adducted, flexed, internal rotated humerus.

come the obstacle presented by joint dysfunction and limitations of motion. Instead of utilizing the necessary range of motion at the joint required to achieve the movement goal, the body involuntarily will need to compromise. This compromise will occur at the accessory movements of the joint, with "trick" and compensatory movements.

For example, a tennis player with a protracted right shoulder girdle must achieve full shoulder extension with horizontal abduction. When there is glenohumeral joint dysfunction, in order to attain this movement goal, the humeral head will sublux anteriorly during the movement, in order to allow the "compromise" to reach the end movement target which requires more range of physiologic extension than available to this tennis player. This "pseudo" extension, achieved via excessive anterior shear of the humeral head, is not within the normal healthy constraints of joint movement. The accessory movements at the joint surface are now pathological, and as a result of this compensation, the glenohumeral joint capsule will become dysfunctional, possibly developing fascial dysfunction at the anterior aspect of the joint capsule, and a tightening of the posterior joint capsule. Assessment is complex. Range of motion should be evaluated while maintaining normal articular balance between the glenoid fossa and the humeral head. For example, gross physiologic extension is measured while evaluating excessive, pathologic anterior glide of the humeral head. The therapist can thus discover the total dysfunctional pattern which requires structural rehabilitation and functional reeducation and training.

Postural dysfunction indicates articular imbalance, joint hypomobility, and limitations in physiological ranges of motion. Manual therapy techniques can be performed at areas of postural dysfunction in order to improve articular balance and increase joint mobility and ranges of physiologic motions. Postural deviations on any and all planes are an indication for treatment.

The general sequence guidelines for manual therapy are as follows:

- Assess postural dysfunction on all three planes: sagittal, coronal, transverse.
- Treat proximal to distal.
- Treat area of greatest postural dysfunction first.
- Treat according to static postural dysfunction first.
- Treat according to dynamic postural dysfunction after static postural dysfunction.

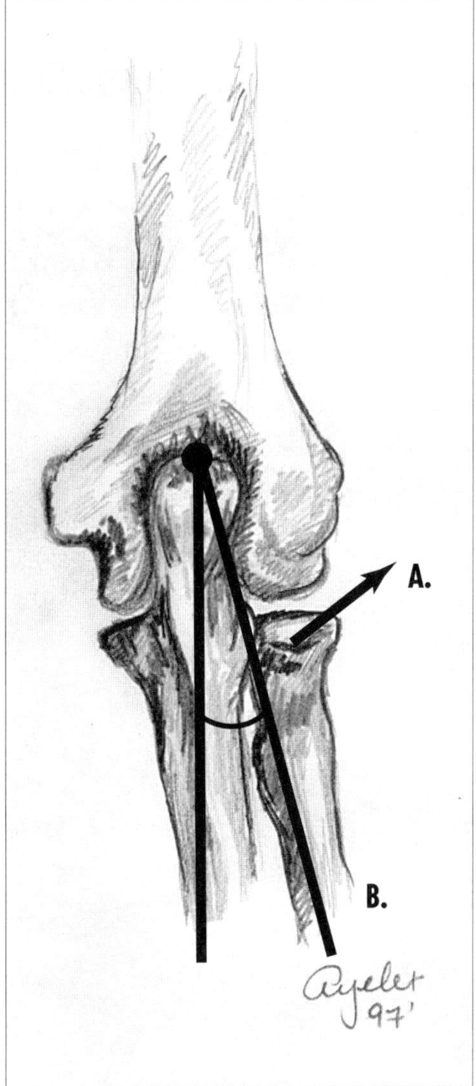

Figure 7. Typical Compensatory Postures: Typical elbow compensations include: **A.** anterior proximal radial head; **B.** abducted ulna and a flexed elbow.

CHAPTER 2

MUSCLE ENERGY AND 'BEYOND' TECHNIQUE

A CONCEPT OF BIOMECHANICS AND THE QUANTUM ENERGETIC FORCES WITHIN THE INTRA-ARTICULAR JOINT SPACES

The Intra-Articular Spaces of Sacral Joints

Treatment of biomechanical dysfunction is not unique. For a long time, many disciplines have attempted to achieve long-lasting effects on joint dysfunction, especially at the lumbosacral junction (L5/S1). The attempts have been unsuccessful, i.e., there does not appear to be one good solution for the tens of thousands of persons affected by low back pain and sciatica. Most spinal surgery occurs at this L5/S1 junction, which reflects that this problem causes significant pain and disability, as well as high cost for health care recipients and taxpayers.

The lumbosacral junction has always been assessed, until recently, for signs of limited mobility. Essentially, L5 at the lumbosacral junction has been assessed like every other spinal segment. This evaluation is not adequate. There is a difference between L5 and other lumbar segments: The lumbosacral junction has reciprocal motion present on three planes, which is not present between L1 through L5.

What is this reciprocal movement at the lumbosacral junction? During sagittal plane motion, the base of sacrum glides in the opposite direction of L5 movement: L5 flexes during posterior sacral glide, and L5 extends during anterior sacral glide. On the transverse plane, L5 rotates to the right while sacrum rotates to the left, and L5 rotates to the left while sacrum rotates to the right. During motion on a coronal plane, there is similar reciprocal motion, i.e., the sacrum side bends in the opposite direction of L5 side bending.

There is a unique concept under investigation by Frank Lowen and (Weiselfish) Giammatteo and others: Problems of sacral biomechanics are in fact problems of the intra-articular spaces. A quantum physics explanation has been developed, explaining why there are limitations of motion at the lumbosacral junction. There is energy within the joint spaces surrounding sacrum, including within the sacroiliac joints, L5 and the sacral base, and between the facets of L5 and S1. There may be a compromise of this energy, which is a disturbance of the quantum energetic forces within the joint spaces. This energy, in the joint spaces around sacrum, presents itself as a uni-planar disturbance within the manifested limitations of motion.

An additional concept, which requires further explanation from a physics perspective, regards "axes." When there is movement which is anterior to midline, the hypothetical axis of motion is positioned anterior to the body part in motion. When there is posterior movement, the axis of motion is positioned behind that body part, where the movement forces are directed. Axes, although conceptual, are forces which are dynamic in nature and reflect motion of moving parts. The direction of the movement is significant; the direction corresponds with the position of the axis on all three planes: sagittal, coronal and transverse.

Sagittal plane movement at the lumbosacral junction is flexion and extension. The movement is different from lumbar spine flexion and extension, because of reciprocal motion. At the lumbosacral junction, when L5 flexes, it is displaced in an antero-inferior direction, while the sacral base glides posterior. Lumbosacral flexion includes both the anterior motion of L5 and the posterior motion of the sacral base. Where is the axis of motion for lumbosacral flexion? Is there a separate anterior axis for L5, with a different posterior axis for S1? This is not reasonable, because lumbosacral flexion is a co-joined motion of L5 together with S1. The axis of motion is neither in front of L5, nor behind S1. The axis of motion for lumbosacral flexion is between L5 and S1, through the disc, with the penetration being midline through the disc. Various phenomena of the L5 disc have been found on dissection. The major part of the disc to be considered appears to be the middle of the nuclear material, which is denser. There are less deviations from midline at the central portion of the disc during movements.

When there is a co-joined motion in the human body between two structures, similar to the motion at the lumbosacral junction, the movement is reflexive in nature. This neuro-reflexogenic-induced capacity for reciprocal motion at the lumboscral junction allows greater movement rather than lesser. Thus, the amount of available motion on any one of the three planes for L5 and S1 is much greater than at any other vertebral segment.

While flexion and extension occur at the lumbosacral junction, movement occurs at both sacroiliac joints. Thus, there must be a co-joined motion capacity of L5/S1 together with the SI joints, which are neuro-reflexogenically able to cooperate with L5 and S1. The sacrospinous ligaments appear to be involved in this participation of cooperated activity.

During torsions of the lumbosacral junction there is also co-joined motion between the lumbosacral junction and bilateral sacroiliac joints. Torsions are the major L5/S1 movement during ambulation. These motions are tri-planar and concomitant on three planes: sagittal, coronal and transverse. When heel strike occurs, there are extension forces affecting the leg in stance phase, which cause a tendency of the sacrum to extend on the side of heel strike. Yet the sacrum cannot extend, because the piriformis is placing an anterior force on the sacrum on that side. The pull of the piriformis will rotate the sacrum towards the side of swing phase, and as the sacrum rotates, side bending of the sacrum occurs to the same side. During midstance, there is a greater force of the piriformis, causing maximal rotation of the sacrum towards the side of mid-swing phase. This end range of rotation will pull the sacrum in a transverse plane posterior on the side of swing phase. The horizontal limb of the articular surface of sacrum accommodates in order to displace sacrum in this manner.

The Forces of Ambulation Through the Intra-Articular Spaces of the Lower Quadrant

During mid-stance towards toe-off there is a transfer of forces from the leg in stance phase towards the leg in swing phase. The extension forces are decreasing throughout mid-stance towards toe-off. While the extension forces decrease, the tendency of the sacrum to extend is eliminated. The piriformis pull is decreased, so the rotation force towards the side of swing phase is reduced. When these rotation forces are reduced, the side bending of sacrum on the side of swing phase decreases. As the forces of rotation towards the swing phase side are reduced, the transverse motion of sacrum on the side of swing phase in a posterior direction subsides. The articular surface of sacrum will no longer be translated on a transverse plane along the horizontal limb of the joint surface. When the forces of extension are eliminated as soon as toe-off occurs, there will be an initiation of momentum-induced forces which affects the leg which is now beginning swing phase. These momentum forces of the body are dependent on energy, the life force, the production of ATP, and metabolic rate. Requirements for momentum-induced motion include muscle fiber strength, recruitment of muscle fibers, neuronal health, and more.

Foot-ground contact occurs during stance phase. This contact is similar to the contact of the wind with water of the ocean. The wind has a force, a velocity, and an amplitude; the water of the ocean transcribes the force. Typically, the evidence of this force occurs on shore, when there could be a tidal wave if the strength of this force, and the amplitude, is intense. When the shore begins to erode, there is an environmental explanation for this erosion. A similar circumstance occurs in the body. When the wind and water meet, there are displacements of energy on three planes. When the foot and ground meet, during standing and ambulation, there are displacements of energy on three planes, which are similar in nature to the displacement of the forces on the water. These forces are transcribed up the leg within the intra-articular spaces. The most significant intra-articular spaces are the tibiotalar, tibiofemoral, and the femoroacetabular spaces. An accommodation to these forces occurs at the sacrum, within the intra-articular joint spaces of the sacroiliac joints and the lumbosacral junction.

The accommodation to foot-ground forces at the sacral joint spaces is a major function of sacrum. The 3-planar forces within the sacral joint spaces, the sacroiliac joints and the lumbosacral junction, are further displaced and transcribed from those joint spaces throughout the body. The forces which converged in the joint spaces of sacrum in a 3-planar manner are now transcribed throughout the joint spaces of the body. These forces are transcribed through the spinal joint spaces, and also through the intra-articular spaces of the soft joints. These soft joints include, for example, the joint spaces between the liver and the diaphragm, between the heart and the pericardium, and between the muscle bellies of different muscles. This transcription of forces occurs between cells and fibers, as well as between those larger structures which have a role in functional organization.

In order that the forces reach the sacrum in a manner that will not cause erosion of the sacral joint surfaces, the lower extremity joints must be aligned, with good articular balance and good joint mobility, and most of all adequate intra-articular joint spaces. The nature of the joint space is similar to the nature of the ocean which is affected by the wind and is able to transcribe the forces of the wind in a manner that will promote healthy shores rather than cause erosion. The intra-articular spaces of the legs are able to transcribe the foot-ground forces in a 3-planar manner, and these forces are transcribed through every joint space (between muscle bellies, between muscle and bone, between blood vessels and muscles, and between cells and fibers). The most significant joint spaces which will determine the quality of forces affecting sacrum are the tibiotalar joint spaces, the tibiofemoral joint space, and the hip joint between the femoral head and the acetabulum.

Muscle Energy and 'Beyond' Technique is an approach to correct the dysfunction of intra-articular spaces, and is taught in Dialogues in Contemporary Rehabilitation courses. The techniques for the lower extremity are goal-oriented, intended to improve the vertical dimensions of the intra-articular joint space. This approach thereby facilitates transcription of foot-ground forces which are transcribed up the leg to the sacral joint spaces for redistribution. The joint spaces of sacrum are treated to accommodate these forces. There is less force within the sacral joint spaces because there is no acceleration (force equals mass times acceleration). The transcription of forces in sitting is similar to the transcription of forces during standing (as compared to the forces during ambulation and running which are characterized by increased amplitude of force as the result of acceleration). The transcription of these sacrum forces and ground forces during sitting has less erosion capacity because the displacement forces on three planes are not as intense. These forces are transcribed through the body's intra-articular spaces. There is an accommodation to these forces within the sacral joint spaces which are then distributed throughout the body.

What is the character of "transcription of forces"? There is a particle and a wave motion of energy which displaces fluids, similar to the displacement of ocean water when the energy of the wind is transcribed on the water towards the shore. This particle and wave-like motion of energy from foot-ground forces and from sacrum-ground contact (i.e., in sitting) requires only space. The fluid, as a medium of transcription, will be more accommodating if it is less viscous and less dense. The more the fluid within the joint spaces is of similar density to water, the more normal the transcription of forces through this medium of fluid can occur.

The upper extremity joints also require intra-articular spaces of perfect alignment and dimension. These spaces are *energetic force torques* for momentum and pressure-displaced and induced motion. When Muscle Energy and 'Beyond' Technique is used to correct the vertical dimensions of the upper extremity intra-articular spaces, the movements are powerful, requiring less strength for more translation and rotation displacement of the arm and trunk.

An interesting concept is the perpetuation of forces through the body. What is the nature of pressure and distance of transcription? How much pressure is required within the joint space? Excessive pressure will apparently inhibit the transcription of these forces through the joint spaces, because of the inherent resistance which pressure provides to energy within an encapsulated area. Too little pressure will be insufficient for medium consistency. Pressure regulation within the joint spaces is important, must be investigated, and often addressed with a person who requires treatment of joint spaces.

Muscle Energy and 'Beyond' Technique reaches inside the joint, beyond the problem of articular balance and joint mobility. Muscle Energy and 'Beyond' Technique is the exceptional therapeutic process which addresses vertical dimension within the joint space. The person is provided a restoration of the system of energy which flows through the joint spaces. This energy rests within the joint spaces for maintenance of vertical dimension. During rest, there is a static particle movement of the energy which flows through the joint spaces, similar to the motion of water molecules in the ocean. During movement there is an increase in the wave-like motion of energy within the joint space, similar to the ocean affected by wind.

Regarding This Book

This book introduces Muscle Energy and 'Beyond' Technique, with thanks to those who contributed foundations for this understanding, including Fred Mitchell, Sr., D.O., Hoover, D.O., Ruddy, D.O., and others. Without their foundation, this approach would not have evolved. This book includes the approach Muscle Energy and 'Beyond' Technique for the peripheral joints of the upper and lower extremities. An approach for pressure normalization within the intra-articular spaces of the legs is introduced. Ambulation facilitation with use of Synchronizers which are reflex governing mechanisms discerned by Lowen and (Weiselfish) Giammatteo is included. The basic techniques for upper and lower extremity normalization of articular balance with Strain and Counterstrain Technique, developed by Lawrence Jones, D.O., is presented. This Strain and Counterstrain approach will correct the Synergic Pattern Imprint in chronic and neurologic clients. The techniques are expected to attain normal joint mobility to improve the accessory movements of the pelvis, leg and arm joints. An introduction to Tendon Release Therapy, and Soft Tissue and Articular Myofascial Release to treat the fascial restrictions of the arms and legs, and to improve capsular and ligamentous tensions, is included. An approach to address complex ligament dysfunction with Ligament Fiber Therapy is introduced. The contents of this book will provide alternatives for the person whose function is inhibited by physical and energetic dysfunction affecting the arms and legs.

Muscle Energy and 'Beyond' Technique: A 3-Planar Approach to Treatment of Intra-Articular Joint Spaces for Energy Distribution and Vertical Dimension

These three concepts are equally important, although there are variables of significance for different clients.

Joint Mobility

The joint mobility of the joint surfaces of any joint is important for movement of that joint. Ranges of motion occur on three planes: sagittal, coronal and transverse. Of course, there is more than just the 3-planar uni-directional and uni-planar movement of a joint. When joint motions are co-joined, in other words when joints cooperate for the production of movement at one joint, there is exceptional joint mobility attained beyond the three planes.

Flexion and extension are uni-directional sagittal plane movements. Abduction and adduction are uni-directional coronal plane movements. External and internal rotations are uni-directional transverse plane movements. Horizontal abduction and horizontal adduction of the glenohumeral joint are also uni-directional movement on a transverse plane, but require the co-joined cooperative movements of the elbow, wrist, hand, and finger joints. The joint mobility of all involved articular surfaces is affected.

The glides of the joint surfaces affect joint mobility. These glides occur because of the pushes and the pulls of muscle fibers which attach to the bones. There are also rotations which occur at the joint surfaces, which are the results of energetic displacement secondary to intersecting forces which are caused by movement. There are approximations which occur at joint surfaces, and distractions that are the result of mechanical pushes and pulls on the joint surface, which are then transduced into energetic displacement.

Palpation of Joint Mobility

It is important to focus on active and passive physiologic ranges of motion as they pertain to joint surface mobility. Perform *assisted active* ranges of motion while palpating accessory joint mobility close to the joint surface of the moving surface. For example, during assisted active shoulder abduction, palpate for smooth caudal glide of the humeral head in the glenoid fossa.

Remember that most *norms* have been measured and documented on average (dysfunctional) bodies. If you question the information in this text as incorrect, please treat your clients in the manner presented in this book. Then reassess. Look for norms.

Accessory Motions: Glides

When the moving surface is convex with the stable and fixed non-moving surface concave (for example the glenohumeral joint), the accessory glides are as follows:

- Flexion: posterior glide
- Extension: anterior glide
- Abduction: caudal glide
- Adduction: superior glide
- External rotation around a vertical axis: anterior glide with distraction
- Internal rotation around a vertical axis: posterior glide with distraction
- Horizontal abduction: anterior glide with approximation
- Horizontal adduction: posterior glide with approximation

When the moving joint surface is concave on a convex fixed and stable joint surface, for example the tibiofemoral (knee) joint, the accessory glides are as follows:

- Flexion: anterior glide
- Extension: posterior glide
- Abduction: medial glide and approximation on the joint side of abduction

- Adduction: lateral glide and approximation on the joint side of adduction
- External rotation: lateral glide
- Internal rotation: medial glide

Joint play is a term used for unlimited motion options within the joint space, passively performed by mechanical pushes and pulls. These motions are not physiologic.

Articular Balance

Articular balance is the relationship of the two articulating joint surfaces from anatomical neutral throughout a full physiologic movement. Articular balance will be viewed from a non-physiologic observation, for example:

- when there is a caudal subluxation of the humeral head in the glenoid fossa, secondary to excessive tone of the latissimus dorsi which depresses the humeral head;
- when there is a lateral tibial shear at the proximal tibial plateau, secondary to an inappropriate balance of ligamentous tension of the ligaments surrounding the knee joint.

When there is faulty articular balance, the two articulating joint surfaces do not maintain normal relationship throughout the range of physiologic movement, resulting in limitations of passive and active ranges of motion. The joint mobility may not be affected, i.e., there may be full glides attained with mobility testing. Long-term problems of articular balance at a joint typically result in capsular tensions which result in joint hypomobility. Joint hypomobility problems which are chronic typically result in ligamentous strains which cause more articular balance problems. It is thus common to discover both joint mobility dysfunction as well as articular balance dysfunction when there are joint problems.

Ligaments are connective tissue. Histologic assessment has discovered different ligament fiber types. One type of fiber appears to be longitudinal, while another type appears to be horizontal. The horizontal or longitudinal orientation of the fibers of the ligaments appears to play an important role. The author hypothesizes, from evidence during clinical research studies, that the longitudinal fibers are for guidance and direction of the distal bone to which the ligament is attached. The horizontal fibers of the ligaments appear to connect the two neighboring bones, in order to provide feedback for proprioception as to whether the two bones are working together in an appropriate manner during resting state and during dynamic motion.

The instability of a joint with ligamentous problems may be more severe for a person than joint hypomobility problems secondary to capsule dysfunction. Both the direction of the moving part, as well as the coordinated activity of the attached two bones will likely be affected with ligament tension problems. This causes instability which may predispose a person more often to injury.

Intra-Articular Space and Vertical Dimension

This is a unique concept which is under clinical investigation by Lowen and (Weiselfish) Giammatteo regarding the system of intra-articular spaces. (Vertical dimension has been discussed often in literature about temporo-mandibular disorders.) The affected system of intra-articular spaces apparently underlies all joint problems, and repercussions associated with dysfunctional intra-articular spaces include capsule dysfunction as well as ligamentous problems. Capsule problems cause joint hypomobility. Ligamentous dysfunction causes loss of articular balance of the joint surfaces.

The spaces within the joints are maintained with energy that has a vibrational molecular particle motion. This energy is entrapped within the fluid of the spaces. When the fluid becomes excessively viscous and dense, the energy does not circulate through the system of intra-articular spaces. The entrapped energy within the intra-articular space will be free for exit and entry as long as there is fluid. This fluid is the synovial fluid within the joint space, which interfaces with the matrix of the connective tissue. When there are increases in the density of this fluid, proteins, long chain fatty acids, and toxins will be trapped inside the joint spaces, as the interstitium is affected. This increase in density affects the metabolism, which includes passage of nutrients into the cells, and also delivery of waste products, including proteins, long chain fatty acids and toxins from the cells into the lymph capillaries. This transport of waste products will be dysfunctional when there is increased viscosity of the fluids. There are lymph nodes in each joint space of each peripheral joint to ensure that the lymph load of waste products is purified, so that these joint spaces are only filled with pure soluble fluid and energy.

When there is dysfunction of the intra-articular space, the total system of energy flow through the body's joint spaces is affected.

Treatment of Biomechanical Dysfunction of the Extremity Joints; Treatment of Joint Hypomobility

Today, there is a recognition of multiple joint mobilization protocols. These procedures were developed by many different professionals, including Stanley Paris, Freddy Kaltenborn, John Mennell, Geoffrey Maitland and others who developed uni-planar musculoskeletal techniques for increasing joint mobility. These approaches were developed to address intra-capsular as well as ligamentous dysfunction. "Capsular patterns" were recognized by professionals who observed consistent variables in their clients' typical manifestation of joint dysfunctions. Often capsular problems were considered ligamentous dysfunctions. The majority of the mobilization procedures were stretch-oriented, although Maitland developed a neurologic-based approach called "painful technique" for treatment of acute joint dysfunction, using very low amplitude oscillation mobilizations.

These mobilization techniques are still used today, and benefit clients with dysfunctions of the capsule, especially when there are adhesions of elasto-collagenous fibers. These direct stretch-like methods are also effective to address intra-articular adhesions. Yet the field of manual therapy is moving towards less direct approaches, looking for decreased resistance from body tissues. Because joint mobility problems are dysfunctions of the capsule, which are fascial problems, fascial release techniques are particularly effective and efficient. The Soft Tissue Myofascial Release Technique, a 3-Planar Fascial Fulcrum approach developed by (Weiselfish) Giammatteo, will correct the majority of problems which are fascial restrictions affecting joint mobility secondary to extra-articular dysfunction. The Articular Fascial Release Technique, a 3-planar approach for correction of capsular and ligamentous adherences, is presented as well in this book. When the joint mobility is compromised because of muscle tension of the sarcomere, i.e., protective muscle spasm, there is a remarkable approach for intervention: Strain and Counterstrain Technique, developed by Lawrence Jones, D.O.

Treatment of Articular Balance Dysfunction

Articular balance is the relationship between two articular surfaces of a joint throughout a full physiologic range of motion. Often there is articular balance dysfunction at rest and during inner ranges of motion. This would be secondary to severe hypertonicity of the muscle fibers attached to the bones of that joint, or due to significant extra-articular or articular fascial restrictions. These articular fascial restrictions may be capsule or ligament. When the articular balance problem is evident only during movement, rather than at rest, the problem surfaces during mid and outer ranges of motion. These problems are less severe, and are also secondary to protective muscle spasm and capsule/ligament dysfunction.

The ligaments are "special." Rather than being totally affected by fascial release techniques, there are other methods for release of ligament tensions which will be presented in this book. The ligaments are a "system." All of the ligaments function together in the body as a whole, but also as units. Their intercommunication system, when they work as a functional complete system, is not yet understood. When any one ligament stretches, all ligaments of the body respond. To attain this response, there must be a neuro-reflexogenic system of communication. This possibly occurs at a spinal reflex level, but must also have higher level neural reflex involvement for this total body response.

Another interesting phenomenon is the longitudinal ligament fibers which function as a single unit for their individual joint, yet also work with all the other longitudinal ligament fibers of the body as a whole. These fibers appear to be responsible for "direction" of movement. The longitudinal fibers are considered by the author as the Guidance System. In comparison, the horizontal fibers of the ligaments do not appear to work together as a total body functional unit, but rather appear to be restricted in function as individual ligament fibers which focus on their own individual joint. These horizontal fibers are apparently the coordinators of motion between the two bony surfaces which they co-join. Coordination appears to be a major function of these horizontal ligament fibers; they coordinate the activities of neighboring bones.

The approach for release of ligamentous tension for guidance and coordination of joints, and for improved articular balance, is included in this text.

Treatment of Decreased Vertical Dimension of Intra-Articular Spaces

This problem, when it affects one joint, affects all the joints of that extremity. Also, when the energy flow is affected in the extremity, total body flow of energy through the intra-articular spaces is compromised. The 3-planar approach for correction of the dysfunctional joint space is Muscle Energy and 'Beyond' Technique, developed by (Weiselfish) Giammatteo. When there is a disturbance of the quantum energetic forces within the joint space, there is a uni-planar presentation of this disturbance. This treatment approach considers the plane of presentation; a "positional diagnosis" is determined; a "treatment position" is assumed to address this presentation; and the treatment technique is performed. The vertical dimension within the joint space can be restored so that ranges of motion are increased.

CHAPTER 3

LAWS OF BIOMECHANICS

UTILIZING MUSCLE ENERGY AND 'BEYOND' TECHNIQUE

Type II 3-Planar Movement Dysfunction Potentials

- Flexion, External Rotation, Abduction
- Flexion, Internal Rotation, Adduction
- Extension, External Rotation, Abduction
- Extension, Internal rotation, Adduction

Co-joined Transverse and Coronal Plane Movements

- External rotation always occurs with abduction.
- Internal rotation always occurs with adduction.

3-Planar Movements Are Type II Movements

- Flexion and extension are sagittal plane movements.
- External and internal rotations are transverse plane movements.
- Abduction and adduction are coronal plane movements.

Laws of Biomechanics

Type I movement is movement in *neutral* (not flexed or extended). Rotation and side bending in neutral occur to opposite sides. This means: right rotation occurs with left side bending in neutral.

Type II movement is movement in *flexion or extension.* Rotation and side bending in flexion or extension occur to the same side. This means: right rotation occurs with right side bending in flexion and extension.

Type II Movement of the Peripheral Joints

The clinical research of the author has provided evidence that peripheral joints have only Type II movement. *There is no Type I movement at the extremity joints.*

Peripheral joints have only Type II movement.

CHAPTER 4

MUSCLE ENERGY AND 'BEYOND' TECHNIQUE FOR THE LOWER EXTREMITIES

TYPE II MOVEMENT DYSFUNCTIONS

Hip Joint

MOVEMENT–HIP JOINT

Hip joints are femoral/acetabular joints. Physiologic movements of the hips are flexion, extension (sagittal plane); abduction, adduction (coronal plane); external rotation, internal rotation (transverse plane).

Direct accessory movements of the femoral head are:

- Anterior glide for extension
- Posterior glide for flexion
- Caudal glide for abduction
- Cephalad glide for adduction
- Anterior glide plus cephalad glide for internal rotation
- Posterior glide plus caudal glide for external rotation

Type II movements occur whenever the hip is flexed or extended. These dysfunctions are:

- Flexed
- Extended

Type II movement dysfunctions are 3-planar torsion dysfunctions. Four possible Type II dysfunctions can occur at the hip (femoral-acetabular) joint:

- Flexed, Adducted, Internal Rotated
- Flexed, Abducted, External Rotated
- Extended, Adducted, Internal Rotated
- Extended, Abducted, External Rotated

**Internal Rotation occurs with Adduction in Type II movement.
External Rotation occurs with Abduction in Type II movement.**

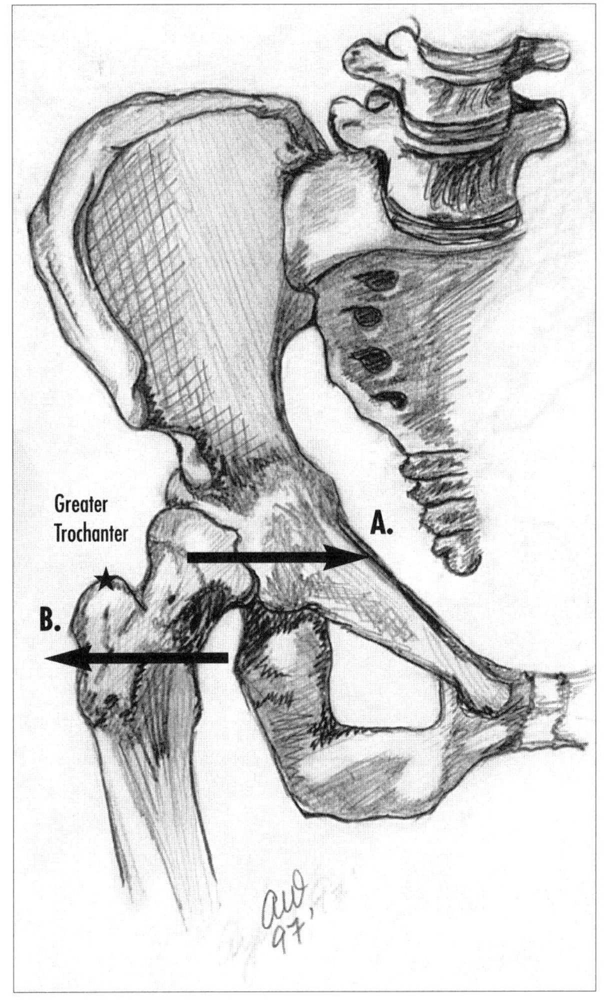

Figure 8. The hip joint is palpated at the greater trochanter for Type II dysfunction. Palpate **A.** medial pull (compression of the femoral head), or **B.** lateral distraction of the femoral head.

ASSESSMENT–HIP JOINT

1. Palpate the glides of the femoral head during physiologic hip flexion and extension.
2. Palpate at the greater trochanter.
3. There should be no approximation or distraction of the femoral head during hip flexion and extension.
4. If the femoral head approximates, there is a medial pull palpated at the greater trochanter.
5. If the femoral head distracts, there is a lateral distraction palpated at the greater trochanter.
6. If the femoral head *approximates,* palpated at the greater trochanter as a medial pull, the hip is stuck *adducted* and *internal rotated.*
7. If the femoral head *laterally distracts,* palpated at the greater trochanter as a lateral distraction, the hip is stuck *abducted* and *external rotated.*
8. If the movement dysfunction is palpated at the greater trochanter *during flexion: the hip cannot flex*, therefore the *hip is stuck extended.*
9. If the movement dysfunction is palpated at the greater trochanter *during extension*: the *hip cannot extend*, therefore the *hip is stuck flexed.*

POSITIONAL DIAGNOSIS–HIP JOINT

EADIR Find in flexion: Extended.

Approximation of femoral head: **AD**ducted, **I**nternally **R**otated

EABER Find in flexion: Extended.

Lateral distraction of femoral head: **AB**ducted, **E**xternally **R**otated

FADIR Find in extension: Flexed.

Approximation of femoral head: **AD**ducted, **I**nternally **R**otated

FABER Find in extension: Flexed.

Lateral distraction of femoral head: **AB**ducted, **E**xternally **R**otated

MOVEMENT BARRIER–HIP JOINT

EADIR Positional diagnosis: Extended, Adducted, and Internally Rotated.

Movement barrier: FABER: Flexion, Abducted, and External Rotation.

EABER Positional diagnosis: Extended, Abducted, and Externally Rotated.

Movement barrier: FADIR: Flexion, Adduction, and Internal Rotation.

FADIR Positional diagnosis: Flexed, Adducted, and Internally Rotated.

Movement barrier: EABER: Extension, Abduction, and External Rotation.

FABER Positional diagnosis: Flexed, Abducted, and Externally Rotated.

Movement barrier: EADIR: Extension, Adduction, and Internal Rotation.

Check the physiologic limitations of motion.

These should correlate with the movement barriers.

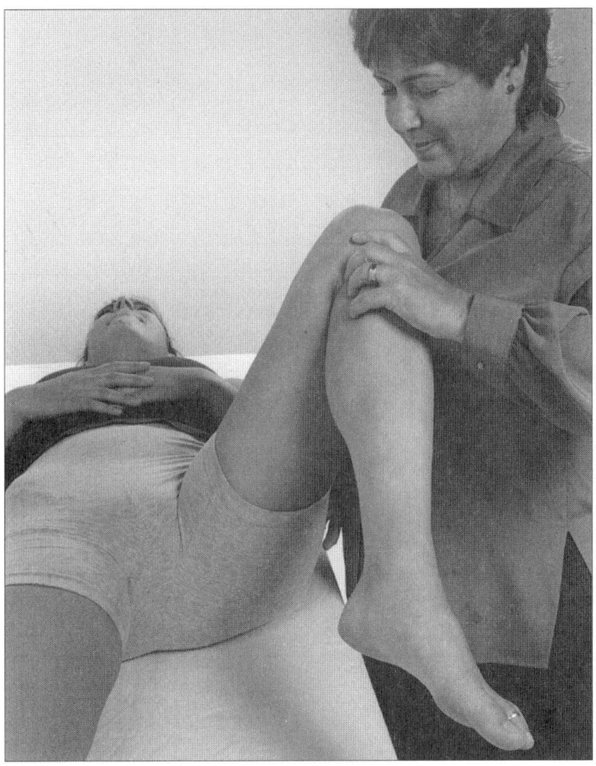

Treatment for EADIR: position in flexion, abduction, external rotation.

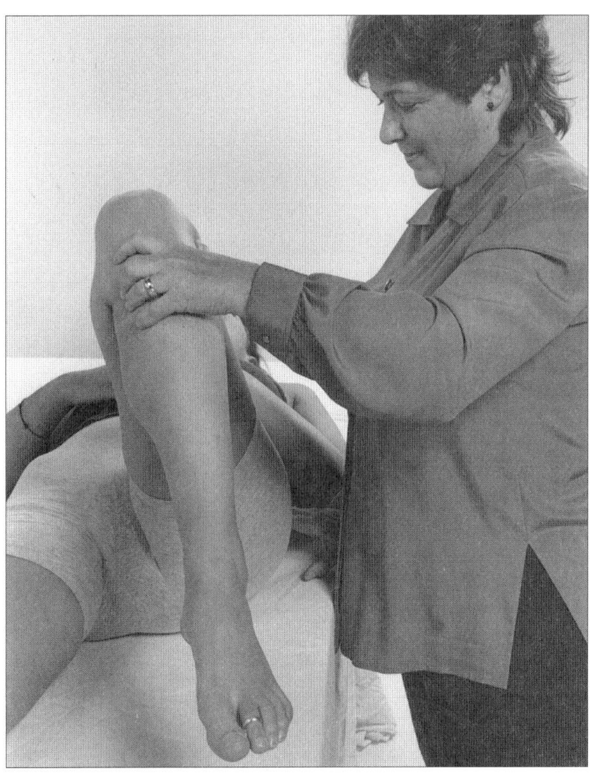

Treatment for EABER: position in flexion, adduction, internal rotation.

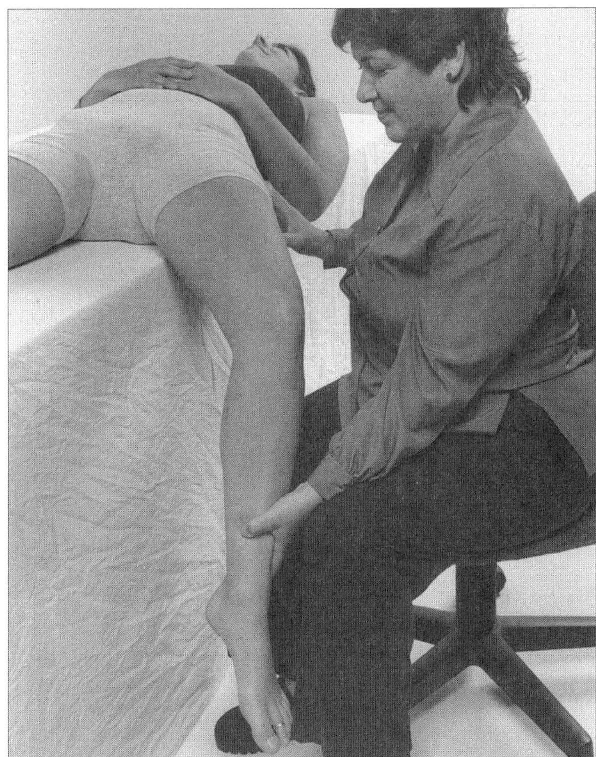

Treatment for FADIR: position in extension, abduction, external rotation.

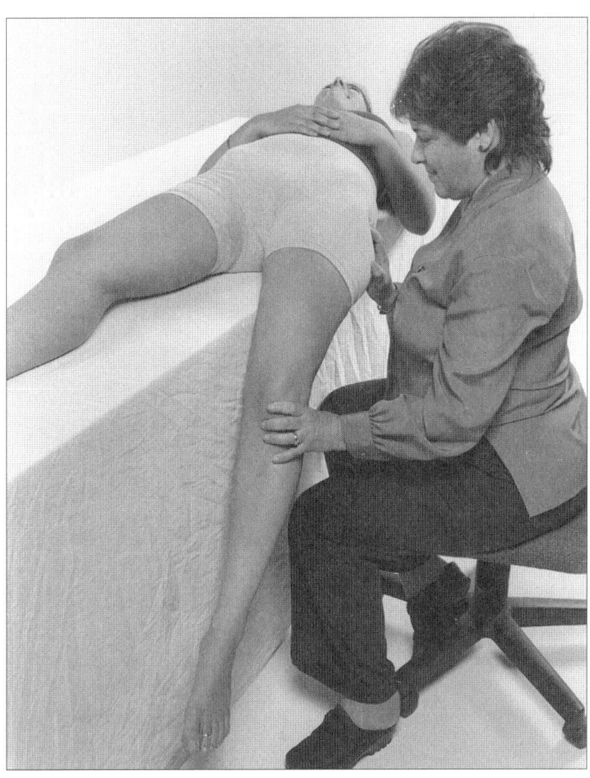

Treatment for FABER: position in extension, adduction, internal rotation.

POSITION OF TREATMENT—HIP JOINT

EADIR Positional diagnosis: Extended, Adducted, and Internally Rotated.

Movement barrier: FABER.

The position of treatment is the same as the movement barrier: FABER: Flex, Abduct, and Externally Rotate the hips to the interbarrier zones. (Note: Refer to Chapter 7.)

EABER Positional diagnosis: Extended, Abducted, and Externally Rotated.

Movement barrier: FADIR.

The position of treatment is the same as the movement barrier: FADIR: Flex, Adduct, and Internally Rotate the hip to the interbarrier zones.

FADIR Positional diagnosis: Flexed, Adducted, and Internally Rotated.

Movement barrier: EABER.

The position of treatment is the same as the movement barrier: EABER: Extend, Abduct, and Externally Rotate the hip to the interbarrier zones.

FABER Positional diagnosis: Flexed, Abducted, and Externally Rotated.

Movement barrier: EADIR.

The position of treatment is the same as the movement barrier: EADIR: Extend, Adduct, and Internally Rotate the hip to the interbarrier zones.

TREATMENT—HIP JOINT

1. Palpate the muscle barrier at the greater trochanter in prone or supine, for extended Type II hip dysfunctions found in flexion. Palpate the muscle barrier at the greater trochanter in prone or supine, for flexed Type II hip dysfunctions found in extension.
2. Move the hip and leg passively to the interbarrier zones on all 3 planes to a 3-planar interbarrier zone.
3. For flexed dysfunctions found in extension: resist any movement of the hip. For extended dysfunctions found in flexion: resist any movement of the hip.
4. Resistance: isometric; 5 grams resistance; 6 seconds resistance; unidirectional/uniplanar resistance.
5. Relaxation.
6. Progress to next 3-planar interbarrier zone.
7. Repetitions: 3.
8. Reassess.

Knee Joint

There are flexed and extended Type II knee joint dysfunctions.

- Physiologic movements of the knee joint include: flexion and extension (sagittal plane).
- Direct accessory movements of the proximal tibial articular surface are:
  1. Anterior glide for extension;
  2. Posterior glide for flexion.
- Lateral glides are dysfunctional if they occur before the last 5 degrees of flexion and extension.
- Rotations are dysfunctional if they occur before the last 5 degrees of flexion and extension.

Type II movements occur whenever the knee joint is:

- Flexed
- Extended

When the knee joint is hyperextended (recurvatum) this is dysfunctional. Normal Type II movements of the knee occur in flexion.

MUSCLE BARRIER–KNEE JOINT

The muscle barrier for assessment of Type II knee dysfunctions can be palpated at the proximal tibial head, on the lateral surface. *Palpate for medial and lateral glides of the proximal tibial head. Lateral glides are more common.*

MOVEMENT–KNEE JOINT

- During flexion, if the proximal tibial head glides laterally, it also externally rotates.
- During flexion, if the proximal tibial head glides medial, it also internally rotates.
- During extension, i.e., when the knee moves from flexed towards anatomic neutral, if the proximal tibial head glides laterally, it also externally rotates.
- During extension, i.e., when the knee moves from flexed towards anatomic neutral, if the proximal tibial head glides medial, it also internally rotates.

APPLICATION

Consider knee joint flexion from anatomic zero to full flexion.
Consider knee joint extension from full flexion to anatomic zero.

Co-joined Transverse and Coronal Plane Movements

External rotation occurs with lateral glide. Internal rotation occurs with medial glide.

Typical Type II knee dysfunction:
Flexed, Lateral Glide, Externally Rotated

Regarding Glides

Glides (medial and lateral) are the modified and natural coronal plane side bending/abduction/adduction motion for the knee.

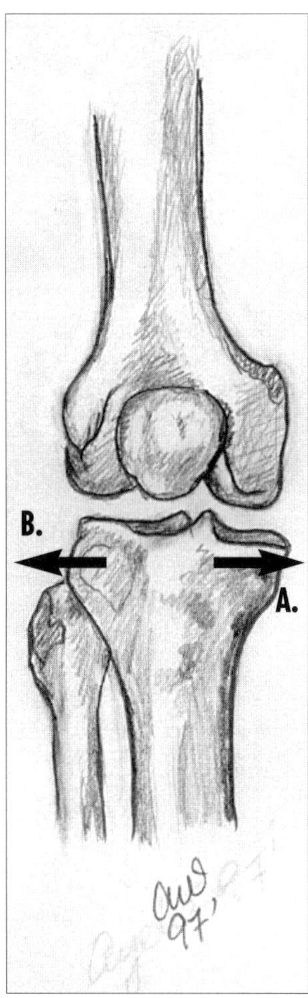

Figure 9. Palpate for **A.** medial glide, or **B.** lateral glide of the proximal tibial head to assess Type II knee joint dysfunction.

ASSESSMENT–KNEE JOINT

In prone (or in supine with lower leg off the bed), assess flexion of the knee joint.

Assess knee joint movement with palpation of the proximal tibial head. Observe if there is lateral or medial glide of the proximal tibial head before the last 5 degrees of end range knee flexion. Lateral glide is modified knee abduction. Medial glide is modified knee adduction. If there is lateral glide of the proximal tibial head, there is also external rotation of the proximal tibial head. If there is medial glide of the proximal tibial head, there is also internal rotation of the proximal tibial head.

In supine, with the leg over the edge of the bed, assess extension of the knee joint.

Assess knee joint movement from full flexion towards a straight leg with palpation of the proximal tibial head. Observe if there is lateral or medial glide of the proximal tibial head before the last 5 degrees of end range knee extension. Lateral glide is modified knee abduction. Medial glide is modified knee adduction. If there is lateral glide of the proximal tibial head, there is also external rotation of the proximal tibial head. If there is medial glide of the proximal tibial head, there is also internal rotation of the proximal tibial head.

POSITIONAL DIAGNOSIS—KNEE JOINT

If dysfunctional glides and rotations occur in knee flexion

- the knee cannot flex;
- the knee is stuck in extension;
- there is an extended Type II knee joint dysfunction.

If dysfunctional glides and rotations occur in knee extension (assessed from full flexion towards a straight knee)

- the knee cannot extend;
- the knee is stuck flexed;
- there is a flexed Type II knee joint dysfunction.

If a lateral glide/external rotation occurs before the last 5 degrees of end-range knee flexion and/or during end-range extension

- the knee is stuck Abducted and Externally Rotated.

If a medial glide/internal rotation occur before the last 5 degrees of end-range knee flexion and/or during end-range extension

- the knee is stuck Adducted and Internally Rotated.

There are four possible Type II knee joint dysfunctions.

FABER Flexed, Abducted, and Externally Rotated
FADIR Flexed, Adducted, and Internally Rotated
EABER Extended, Abducted, and Externally Rotated
EADIR Extended, Adducted, and Internally Rotated

The most common Type II knee joint dysfunction is: FABER.

MOVEMENT BARRIER—KNEE JOINT

FABER The knee is stuck Flexed, Abducted (lateral glide), and Externally Rotated.

Movement barrier: EADIR: the knee cannot Extend, Adduct (glide medial), and Internally Rotate.

FADIR The knee is stuck Flexed, Adducted (medial glide), and Internally Rotated.

Movement barrier: EABER: the knee cannot Extend, Abduct (glide lateral), and Externally Rotate.

EABER The knee is stuck Extended, Abducted (lateral glide), and Externally Rotated.

Movement barrier: FADIR: the knee cannot Flex, Adduct (glide medial), and Internally Rotate.

EADIR The knee is stuck Extended, Adducted (medial glide), and Internally Rotated.

Movement barrier: FABER: the knee cannot Flex, Abduct (glide lateral), and Externally Rotate.

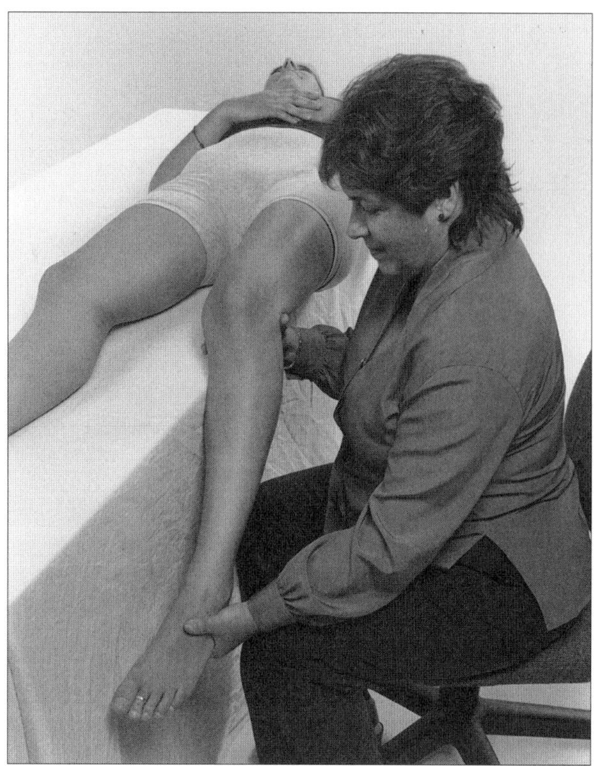

Treatment for FABER: position in extending, adduction, internal rotation.

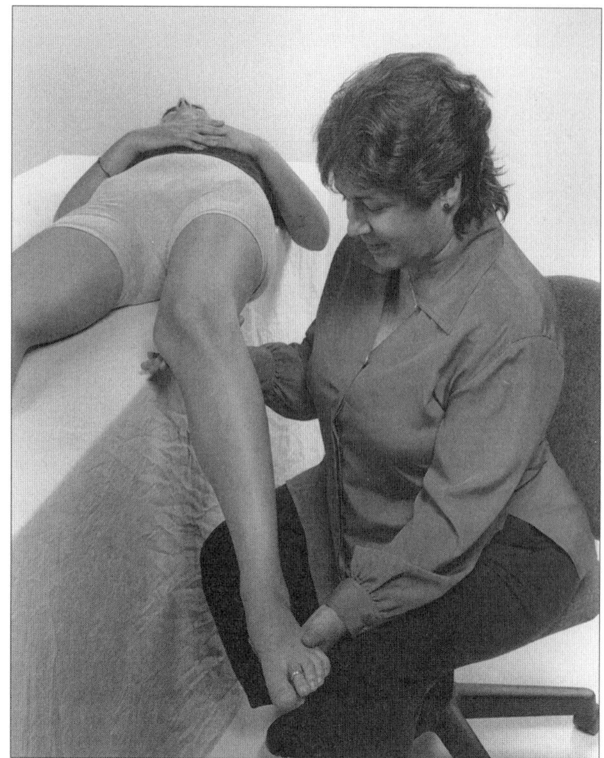

Treatment for FADIR: position in extending, abduction, external rotation.

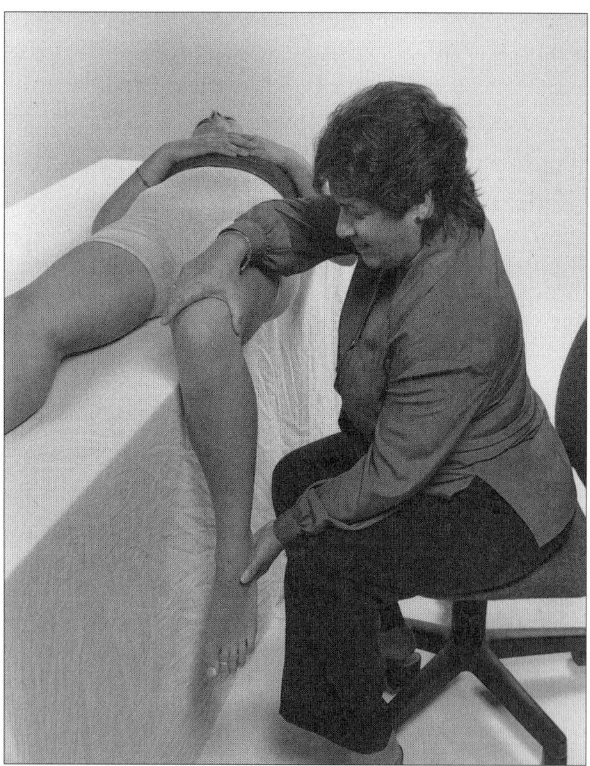

Treatment for EABER: position in flexion, adduction, internal rotation.

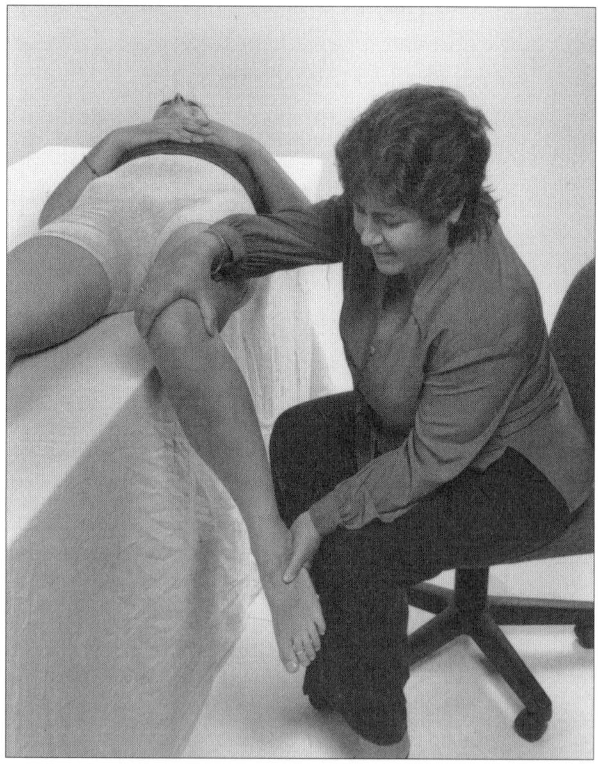

Treatment for EADIR: position in flexion, abduction, external rotation.

POSITION OF TREATMENT–KNEE JOINT

FABER Positional diagnosis: Flexed, Abducted (lateral glide), and Externally Rotated.

Movement barrier: EADIR.

The position of treatment is the same as the movement barrier: EADIR: Extend, Adduct, and Internally Rotate the knee to the interbarrier zones.

FADIR Positional diagnosis: Flexed, Adducted (medial glide), and Internally Rotated.

Movement barrier: EABER.

The position of treatment is the same as the movement barrier: EABER: Extend, Abduct, and Externally Rotate the knee to the interbarrier zones.

EABER Positional diagnosis: Extended, Abducted (lateral glide), and Externally Rotated.

Movement barrier: FADIR.

The position of treatment is the same as the movement barrier: FADIR: Flex, Adduct, and Internally Rotate the knee to the interbarrier zones.

EADIR Positional diagnosis: Extended, Adducted, and Internally Rotated.

Movement barrier: FABER.

The position of treatment is the same as the movement barrier: FABER: Flex, Abduct (put in lateral glide), and Externally Rotate the knee to the interbarrier zones.

TREATMENT–KNEE JOINT

1. Treat flexed Type II knee joint dysfunctions in prone or in supine with knee off the bed, keep hip aligned in neutral (not abducted, not rotated).
2. Treat extended Type II knee joint dysfunctions in prone or in supine with knee off the bed, keep hip aligned in neutral (not abducted, not rotated).
3. Palpate for the muscle barrier at the proximal tibial head. Focus on the lateral aspect of the tibial head.
4. Move the lower leg passively on all 3 planes to a 3-planar interbarrier zone. Can do lateral glide instead of abduction. Can do medial glide instead of adduction.
5. For flexed dysfunctions, move into extension. For extended dysfunctions, move into flexion.
6. Resist knee extension or knee flexion.
7. Resistance: isometric; 5 grams resistance; unidirectional/uniplanar resistance; 6 seconds resistance.
8. Relaxation.
9. Progress to next 3-planar interbarrier zone.
10. Repetitions: 3.
11. Reassess.

Ankle (Tibiotalar) Joint

This joint requires slightly different orientation, since it is dependent on the subtalar (talo-calcaneal) joint for mobility and articular balance. The subtalar joint frequently has intra-articular adhesions. There is no effective Muscle Energy and 'Beyond' Technique for the subtalar (talo-calcaneal) joint. Manipulation and Strain and Counterstrain and Mobilization are effective approaches for the subtalar joint. The most effective and efficient technique for treating subtalar and tibiotalar joint fascial restrictions is "The Secret of the Tibiotalar and Subtalar Joint" Technique (This technique is written up in this text). Prior to, or after, treatment of Type II tibiotalar joint dysfunction, treat the subtalar joint to restore mobility and articular balance.

- Dorsiflexion is always limited; there is never limitation of plantar flexion.
- Dorsiflexion limitations are Extended Type II dysfunctions of the tibiotalar joint. The ankle is stuck plantar flexed (extended). The ankle cannot flex (dorsiflex).
- The positional diagnosis is always *extended.*
- Inversion is adducted. Eversion is abducted.
- Inversion occurs with internal rotation.
- Eversion occurs with external rotation.

ASSESSMENT–ANKLE JOINT

1. Assess movement barrier at the superior surface of talus at the ankle mortise.
2. A lateral glide of talus occurs during internal rotation and adduction. A medial glide of talus occurs during external rotation and abduction.

POSITIONAL DIAGNOSIS–ANKLE JOINT

The Type II torsion patterns of the tibiotalar joint will be:

EADIR Extended, Adducted, and Internally Rotated

EABER Extended, Abducted, and Externally Rotated

The most common ankle joint dysfunction is EADIR.

MOVEMENT BARRIER–ANKLE JOINT

EADIR The tibiotalar joint is stuck: Extended (plantar flexed), Adducted, and Internally Rotated (inverted).

Movement barrier: FABER: The ankle joint cannot Flex (dorsiflex), Abduct, and Externally Rotate (evert).

EABER The tibiotalar joint is stuck Extended (plantar flexed), Abducted, and Externally Rotated (everted).

Movement barrier: FADIR: The ankle joint cannot Flex (dorsiflex), Adduct, and Internally Rotate (invert).

POSITION OF TREATMENT–ANKLE JOINT

EADIR Positional diagnosis: Extended, (plantar flexed), Adducted, and Internally Rotated.

Movement barrier: FABER.

The position of treatment is the same as the movement barrier: FABER: Flex (dorsiflex), Abduct, and Externally Rotate the tibiotalar joint to the interbarrier zones.

EABER Positional diagnosis: Extended (plantar flexed), Abducted, and Externally Rotated.

Movement barrier: FADIR.

The position of treatment is the same as the movement barrier: FADIR: Flex, (dorsiflex), Adduct, and Internally Rotate the tibiotalar joint to the interbarrier zones.

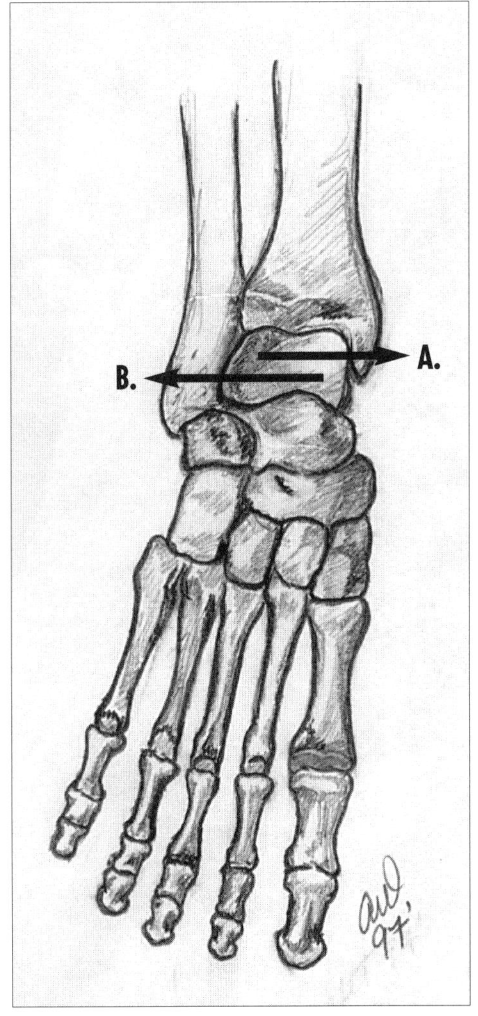

Figure 10. A. Medial glide of talus occurs during internal rotation and adduction of Type II tibiotalar joint dysfunction. **B.** Lateral glide of talus occurs during external rotation and abduction of Type II tibiotalar joint dysfunction.

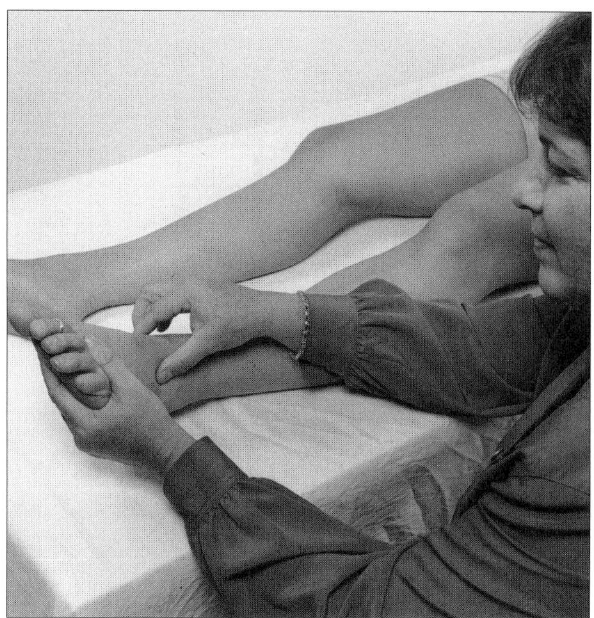
Treatment for EADIR: position in dorsiflexion, abduction, external rotation

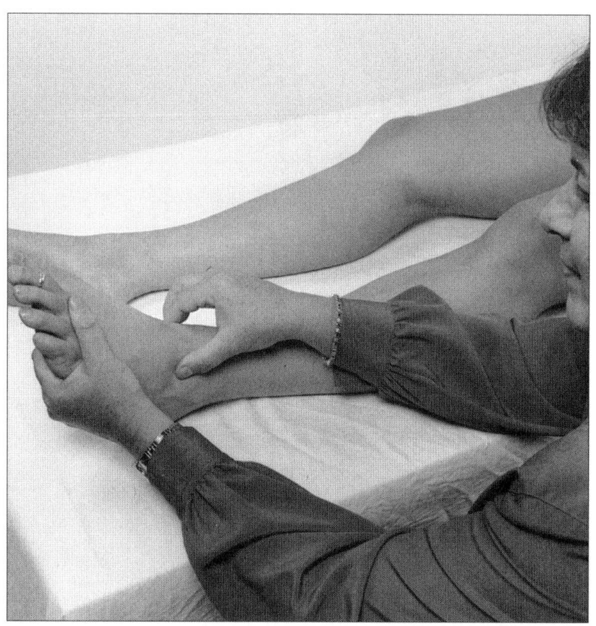
Treatment for EABER: position in dorsiflexion, adduction, internal rotation.

TREATMENT–ANKLE JOINT

1. Treat in supine: Dorsiflexion is the sagittal plane movement.
2. Palpate the movement barrier at the mortise: Observe lateral and medial glides of the superior surface of talus. A lateral glide occurs during adduction and internal rotation. A medial glide occurs during abduction and external rotation.
3. Move the ankle passively in all 3 planes to the 3-planar interbarrier zone.
4. Resist dorsiflexion or plantar flexion.
5. Resistance: Isometric; 5 grams force; unidirectional/uniplanar resistance; 6 seconds resistance.
6. Relaxation.
7. Progress to new 3-planar interbarrier zone.
8. Repetitions: 3.
9. Reassess.

"The Secret of the Tibotalar and Subtalar Joint" Technique

Compression syndromes were first recognized by (Weiselfish) Giammatteo in 1993 as protective modes, similar to protective muscle spasm. The compression syndromes for the tibiotalar joint and the subtalar joint were developed in 1994.

The Tibiotalar Joint Technique

INDICATION

Decreased ankle dorsiflexion.

POSITION

The client is supine, with good neutral alignment of the leg. This means there is anatomic neutral maintained at the hip, knee and ankle. There is 0 degrees coronal plane (hip abduction or adduction); 0 degrees transverse plane (hip internal or external rotation); 0 degrees sagittal plane (hip flexion or extension). Sagittal plane at the knee is 0 degrees (flexion or extension). The ankle is loose packed, without any approximation or distraction at the tibiotalar or subtalar joints.

TREATMENT

1. The practitioner uses both hands, specifically the web spaces. One web space encompasses the anterior aspect of the distal end of the tibia. The other web space encompasses the superior/anterior aspect of the talus. Maintaining good contact throughout the technique is important. There should be minimal "forceful" grip.
2. Both web spaces push on the bony contacts on the following directions simultaneously: posterior and lateral. This means that distal tibia is maintained in a posterior plus a lateral glide, while the talus is maintained in a posterior plus a lateral glide.
3. There will be a lot of "unwinding" which means a tissue tension change. This technique is a "fulcrum" technique. Throughout the duration of the technique, these pressures of posterior plus lateral glide are maintained. No physiologic motion (i.e., flexion, extension, abduction, adduction, or internal/external rotation) is permitted throughout the duration of the technique.

THE RELEASE

The technique will be "completed" when there is no remaining evidence of tissue tension changes in the soft tissues of the leg. For mild problems, the technique may last 3 to 5 minutes. For severe problems, the technique may last up to 10 minutes. Usually, this technique does not take longer than 10 minutes. The nature of the ankle joint problem, together with the severity and chronicity, determine whether the problem is mild, moderate, or severe.

EXPECTED OUTCOME

Ankle dorsiflexion should increase to 75 percent of normal.

The Subtalar Joint Technique

INDICATION

Decreased ankle dorsiflexion.

POSITION

The client is supine, with good neutral alignment of the leg. This means there is anatomic neutral maintained at the hip, knee and ankle. There is 0 degrees coronal plane (hip abduction or adduction); 0 degrees transverse plane (hip internal or external rotation); 0 degrees sagittal plane (hip flexion or extension). Sagittal plane at the knee is 0 degrees (flexion or extension). The ankle is loose packed, without any approximation or distraction at the tibiotalar or subtalar joints.

TREATMENT

1. The practitioner uses both hands. One hand pulls the calcaneus in a longitudinal distraction from the talus. The second hand, thumb and second/third digits, perform a "separation/distraction" between talus and the medial cuneiform. Maintaining good contact throughout the technique is important. There should be minimal "forceful" grip.
2. There will be a lot of "unwinding" which means tissue tension changes. This technique is a "fulcrum" technique. Throughout the duration of the technique, these pressures of "separation/distraction" are maintained. No physiologic motion (i.e., flexion, extension, abduction, adduction, internal/external rotation) is permitted throughout the duration of the technique.

THE RELEASE

The technique will be "completed" when there is no remaining evidence of tissue tension changes in the soft tissues of the leg. For mild problems, the technique may last 3 to 5 minutes. For severe problems, the technique may last up to 10 minutes. Usually, this technique does not take longer than 10 minutes. The nature of the ankle joint problem, together with the severity and chronicity, determine whether the problem is mild, moderate, or severe.

EXPECTED OUTCOME

When the subtalar joint technique is performed after the tibiotalar joint technique, ankle dorsiflexion should increase to 90 percent of normal range of motion.

INTEGRATIVE MANUAL THERAPY

The results of these two techniques are long lasting. A protocol for severe ankle sprain, with resistance to normalization of full dorsiflexion, can include:

1. Tibiotalar Joint Compression Syndrome Technique (see page 29) for mobilization and distraction of the tibiotalar joint.
2. Subtalar Joint Compression Syndrome Technique (see above) for mobilization and distraction of the subtalar joint.
3. Jones Strain and Counterstrain Extended Ankle Technique, to decrease protective muscle spasm of the medial calcaneus.
4. (Weiselfish) Giammatteo's Tendon Release Therapy for the Achilles Tendon.

CHAPTER 5

MUSCLE ENERGY AND 'BEYOND' TECHNIQUE FOR THE UPPER EXTREMITIES

TYPE II MOVEMENT DYSFUNCTIONS

Shoulder (Glenohumeral) Joint

The physiologic movements of the shoulder joint are: flexion, extension (sagittal plane); abduction, adduction (coronal plane); external rotation, internal rotation (transverse plane).

Direct accessory movements of the humeral head are:

- Anterior glide for extension
- Posterior glide for flexion
- Caudal glide for abduction
- Cephalad glide (to neutral) for adduction (from abduction)
- Anterior glide plus caudal glide for internal rotation
- Posterior glide plus cephalad glide for external rotation
- Anterior glide for horizontal adduction
- Posterior glide for horizontal abduction

Note: The literature does not present these movements as "norms." Yet with this therapy, these motions are restored.

Type II movements occur whenever the shoulder is flexed or extended. Type II dysfunctions are:

- Flexed
- Extended

Type II movement dysfunctions are 3-planar torsion dysfunctions. Four possible Type II dysfunctions can occur at the shoulder (glenohumeral) joint:

- Flexed, Adducted, Internal Rotated
- Flexed, Abducted, External Rotated
- Extended, Adducted, Internal Rotated
- Extended, Abducted, External Rotated

Internal Rotation occurs with Adduction in Type II movement. External Rotation occurs with Abduction in Type II movement.

ASSESSMENT–SHOULDER JOINT

1. Palpate the glides of the humeral head during physiologic shoulder flexion and extension.
2. Palpate at the greater tuberosity.
3. There should not be any approximation nor any distraction of the humeral head during shoulder flexion and extension.
4. If the humeral head approximates, there is a medial pull palpated at the greater tuberosity.
5. If the humeral head distracts, there is a lateral distraction palpated at the greater tuberosity.
6. If the humeral head approximates, palpated at the greater tuberosity as a medial pull, the shoulder is stuck adducted and internally rotated.
7. If the humeral head laterally distracts, palpated at the greater tuberosity as a lateral distraction, the shoulder is stuck abducted and external rotated.
8. If the movement dysfunction is palpated at the greater tuberosity during flexion: The shoulder cannot flex, therefore, the shoulder is stuck extended.
9. If the movement dysfunction is palpated at the greater tuberosity during extension: The shoulder cannot extend, therefore, the shoulder is stuck flexed.

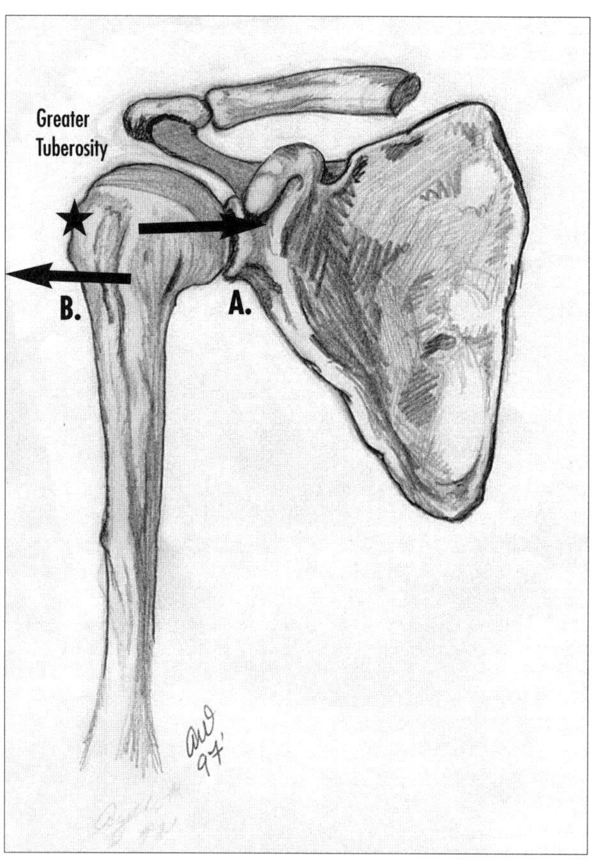

Figure 11. Palpate at the greater tuberosity for Type II dysfunctions of the glenohumeral joint. **A.** Approximation of the humeral head indicates adduction and internal rotation. **B.** Lateral distraction of the humeral head reflects abduction and external rotation.

POSITIONAL DIAGNOSIS–SHOULDER JOINT

EADIR Find in flexion: **E**xtended.

Approximation of humeral head: **AD**ducted, **I**nternally **R**otated.

EABER Find in flexion: **E**xtended.

Lateral distraction of the humeral head: **AB**ducted, **E**xternally **R**otated.

FADIR Find in extension: **F**lexed.

Approximation of the humeral head: **AD**ducted, **I**nternally **R**otated.

FABER Find in extension: **F**lexed.

Lateral distraction of the humeral head: **AB**ducted, **E**xternally **R**otated.

MOVEMENT BARRIER–SHOULDER JOINT

EADIR Positional diagnosis: Extended, Adducted, and Internally Rotated.

Movement barrier: FABER: Flexion, Abducted, and External Rotation.

EABER Positional diagnosis: Extended, Abducted, and Externally Rotated.

Movement barrier: FADIR: Flexion, Adduction, and Internal Rotation.

FADIR Positional diagnosis: Flexed, Adducted, and Internally Rotated.

Movement barrier: EABER: Extension, Abduction, External Rotation.

FABER Positional diagnosis: Flexed, Abducted, and Externally Rotated.

Movement barrier: EADIR: Extension, Adduction, and Internal Rotation.

Check the physiologic limitations of motion. These should correlate with the movement barriers.

POSITION OF TREATMENT–SHOULDER JOINT

EADIR Positional diagnosis: Extended, Adducted, and Internally Rotated.

Movement barrier: FABER.

The position of treatment is the same as the movement barrier: FABER: Flex, Abduct, and Externally Rotate the shoulders to the interbarrier zones.

EABER Positional diagnosis: Extended, Abducted, and Externally Rotated.

Movement barrier: FADIR.

The position of treatment is the same as the movement barrier: FADIR: Flex, Adduct, and Internally Rotate the shoulder to the interbarrier zones.

FADIR Positional diagnosis: Flexed, Adducted, and Internally Rotated.

Movement barrier: EABER.

The position of treatment is the same as the movement barrier: EABER: Extend, Abduct, and Externally Rotate the shoulder to the interbarrier zones.

FABER Positional diagnosis: Flexed, Abducted, and Externally Rotated.

Movement barrier: EADIR.

The position of treatment is the same as the movement barrier: EADIR: Extend, Adduct, and Internally Rotate the shoulder to the interbarrier zones.

TREATMENT–SHOULDER JOINT

1. Palpate the muscle barrier at the greater tuberosity in prone or supine, for extended Type II shoulder dysfunctions found in flexion. Palpate the muscle barrier at the greater tuberosity in prone or supine, for flexed Type II shoulder dysfunctions found in extension.
2. Move the shoulder and arm passively to the interbarrier zone on all 3 planes to a 3-planar interbarrier zone.
3. For flexed dysfunctions found in extension: Resist any movement of the shoulder.
   For extended dysfunctions found in flexion: Resist any movement of the shoulder.
4. Resistance: isometric; 5 grams resistance; unidirectional/uniplanar resistance; 6 seconds resistance.
5. Relaxation.
6. Progress to next 3-planar interbarrier zone.
7. Repetitions: 3.
8. Reassess.

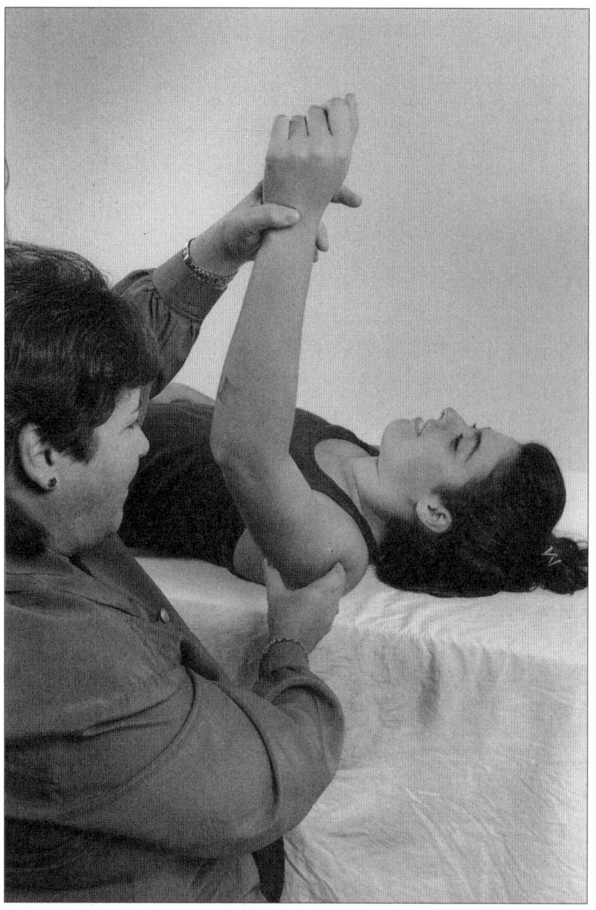

Treatment for EADIR: position in flexion, abduction, external rotation.

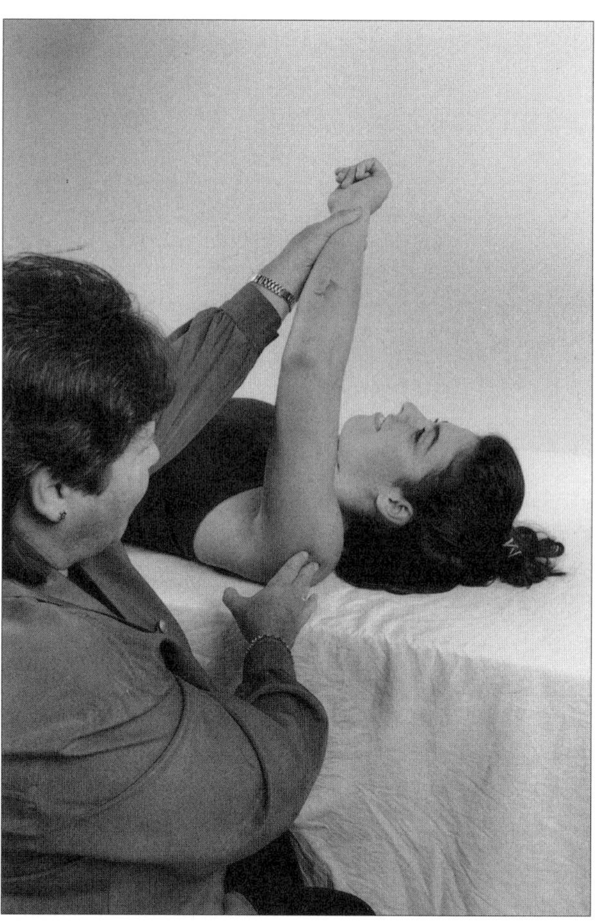

Treatment for EABER: position in flexion, adduction, internal rotation.

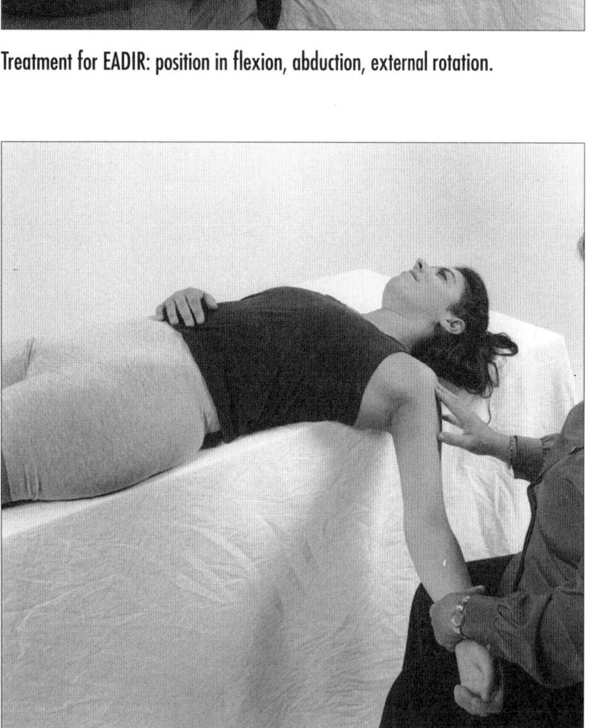

Treatment for FADIR: position in extension, abduction, external rotation.

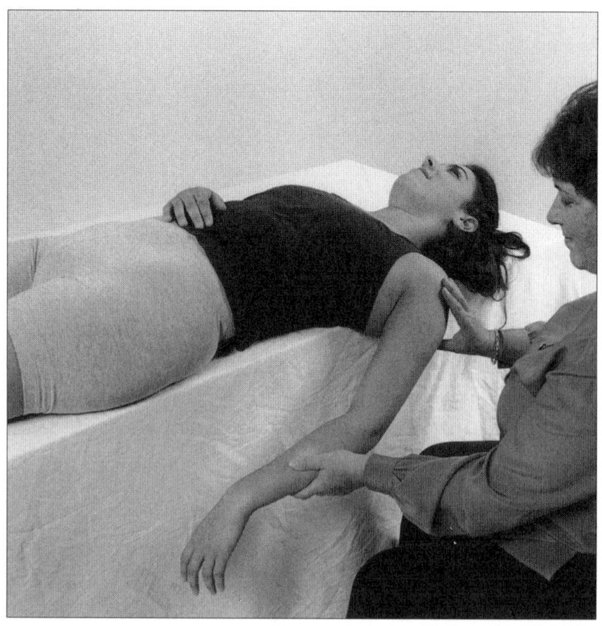

Treatment for FABER: position in extension, adduction, internal rotation.

Sternoclavicular Joint

This joint is a modified physiologic joint. Direct accessory movements are:

- Caudal glide of the clavicular head during abduction of the shoulder;
- Anterior glide of the clavicular head during extension of the shoulder;
- Rotation (superior/posterior) of the clavicular head during flexion of the shoulder;
- Compression/approximation of the clavicular head during horizontal adduction of the shoulder;
- Distraction of the clavicular head during horizontal abduction of the shoulder.
- Internal and external rotations are minimally affected/affect the sternoclavicular joint; these movements are focused at the acromioclavicular joint.

MOVEMENT—STERNOCLAVICULAR JOINT

- Abduction and lateral distraction occur together.
- Adduction and approximation occur together.
- Flexed has two possible Type II variations:
  Abduction and lateral distraction
  Adduction and approximation
- Extended has two possible Type II variations:
  Abduction and lateral distraction
  Adduction and approximation

There are four possible Type II dysfunctions that can occur at the sternoclavicular joint:

- Flexed, Abducted, Lateral Distracted
- Flexed, Adducted, Approximated
- Extended, Abducted, Lateral Distracted
- Extended, Adducted, Approximated

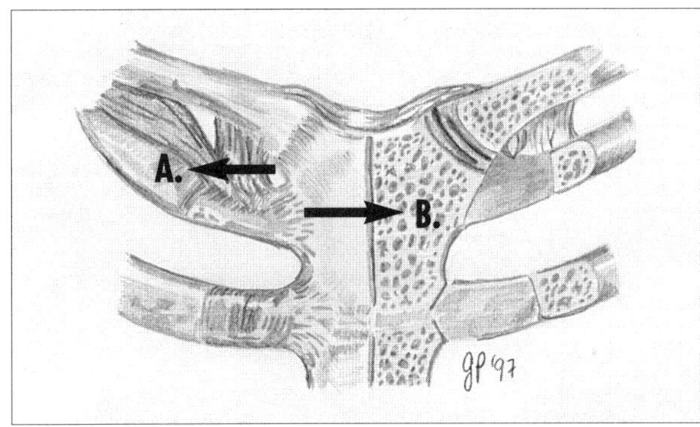

Figure 12. A. Lateral distraction of the proximal clavicle head occurs with abduction. **B.** Approximation of the proximal clavicle head occurs with adduction.

ASSESSMENT—STERNOCLAVICULAR JOINT

1. Palpate the movement barrier at the proximal head of clavicle.
2. Assess: lateral distraction and approximation.
3. Lateral distraction occurs with abduction.
4. Approximation occurs with adduction.

POSITIONAL DIAGNOSIS—STERNOCLAVICULAR JOINT

FABLD Find in extension: Flexed

Lateral distraction of proximal head of clavicle: **AB**ducted, **L**ateral **D**istracted

FADA Find in extension: Flexed

Approximation of proximal head of clavicle: **AD**ducted, **A**pproximated

EABLD Find in flexion: Extended

Lateral distraction of proximal head of clavicle: **AB**ducted, **L**ateral **D**istracted

EADA Find in flexion: Extended

Approximation of proximal head of clavicle: **AD**ducted, **A**pproximated

MOVEMENT BARRIER—STERNOCLAVICULAR JOINT

FABLD The sternoclavicular joint is stuck Flexed (superior/posterior rotation), Abducted, and Lateral Distracted.

Movement barrier: EADA: Extension, Adduction, and Approximation.

FADA The sternoclavicular joint is stuck Flexed (superior/posterior rotation), Adducted, and Approximated.

Movement barrier: EABLD: Extension, Abduction, and Lateral Distraction.

EABLD The sternoclavicular joint is stuck Extended (anterior glide), Abducted, and Lateral Distracted.

Movement barrier: FADA: Flexion, Adduction, and Approximation.

EADA The sternoclavicular joint is stuck Extended, Adducted, and Approximated.

Movement barrier: FABLD: Flexion, Abduction, and Lateral Distraction.

POSITION OF TREATMENT—STERNOCLAVICULAR JOINT

FABLD Extend the arm off the edge of the table until the movement barrier (approximation) is palpated at the proximal clavicle head. Then adduct clavicle and approximate the proximal clavicle head. Position at a 3-planar interbarrier zone.

FADA Extend the arm off the edge of the table until the movement barrier (lateral distraction) is palpated at the proximal clavicle head. Then abduct clavicle and laterally distract the proximal clavicle head. Position at a 3-planar interbarrier zone.

EABLD Flex the arm until the movement barrier (approximation) is palpated at the proximal clavicle head. Then adduct clavicle and approximate the proximal clavicle head. Position at a 3-planar interbarrier zone.

EADA Flex the arm until the movement barrier (approximation) is palpated at the proximal clavicle head. Then abduct clavicle and laterally distract the proximal clavicle head. Position at a 3-planar interbarrier zone.

TREATMENT—STERNOCLAVICULAR JOINT

To position the arm/shoulder to assess movement barriers, and for treatment, follow the following procedures:

1. For flexed sternoclavicular joint dysfunction: In supine; shoulder off edge of the bed; straight arm; no abduction or rotation; passively move into extension.
2. For extended sternoclavicular joint dysfunction: In supine; straight arm; no abduction/adduction or rotation. Passively move into flexion.
3. For abducted and lateral distracted sternoclavicular joint dysfunction: Use fingers on proximal clavicle head. Adduct the clavicle by bringing distal clavicle caudal, and compress the proximal clavicle head towards the manubrium articular surface.
4. For adducted and approximated sternoclavicular joint dysfunction: Use fingers on proximal clavicle head. Abduct the clavicle by bringing distal clavicle superior, and distract the proximal clavicle head away from the manubrium articular surface.
5. Resistance: isometric; 5 grams force; unidirectional/uniplanar resistance; 6 seconds resistance.
6. Relaxation.
7. Repetitions: 3.
8. Reassess.

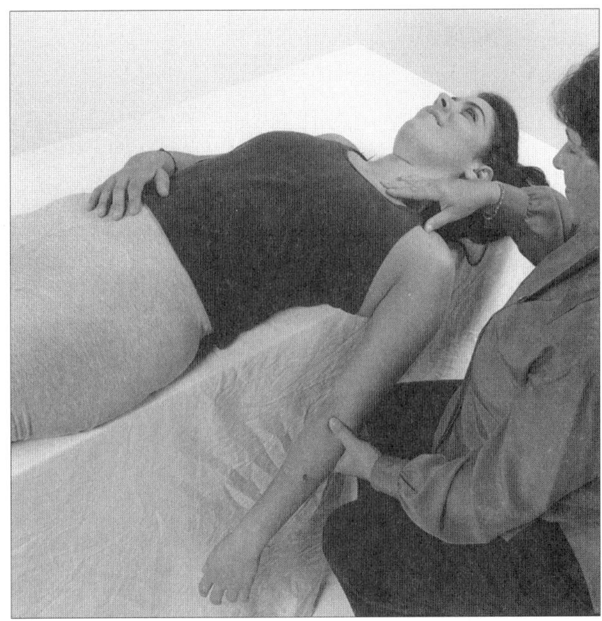

Treatment for FABLD: Extend the arm. Adduct the clavicle. Approximate the head of clavicle.

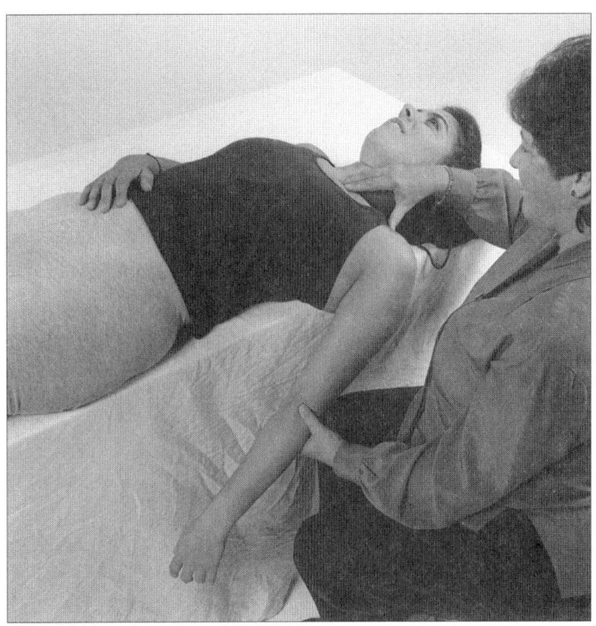

Treatment for FADA: Extend the arm. Abduct the clavicle. Lateral distract the head of clavicle.

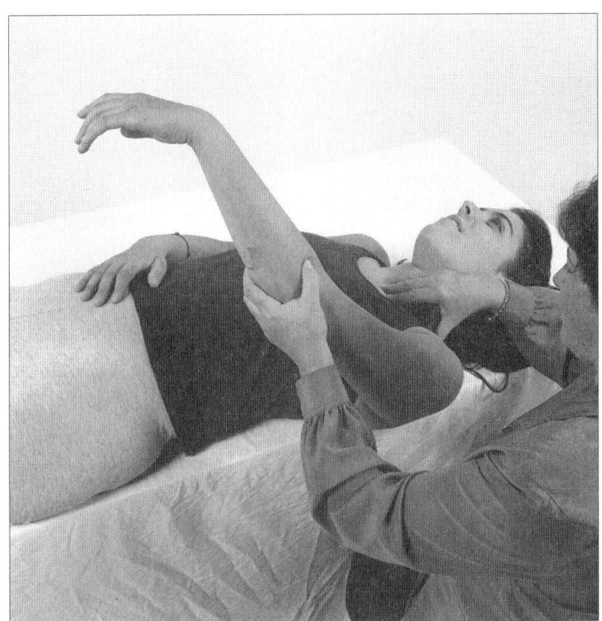

Treatment for EABLD: Flex the arm. Adduct the clavicle. Approximate the head of clavicle.

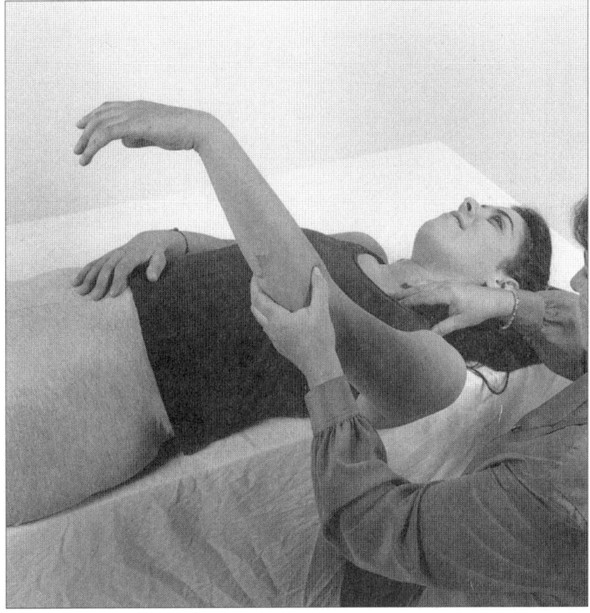

Treatment for EADA: Flex the arm. Abduct the clavicle. Lateral distract the head of clavicle.

Scapulothoracic Joint

The scapulothoracic joint is a pseudo-joint without biomechanical primary dysfunction. Effective treatment for mobility and articular balance of the scapulothoracic joint is attained with: Strain and Counterstrain, Mobilization, Visceral Mobilization, and Myofascial Release.

Acromioclavicular Joint

This joint does not respond well to Muscle Energy and 'Beyond' Technique philosophy. Excellent articular balance and mobility can be attained with Strain and Counterstrain: use the Anterior Acromioclavicular Joint Tender Point and the Jones' Posterior Acromioclavicular Joint Tender Point.

Elbow Joints

The elbow has three joints:

1. Proximal Radioulnar
2. Radiohumeral
3. Humeroulnar

When the elbow joints are treated in this sequence (as above), the Muscle Energy and 'Beyond' Technique is extremely effective and efficient to restore joint mobility, articular balance, and intra-articular space vertical dimension.

The Proximal Radioulnar Joint

ASSESSMENT–PROXIMAL RADIOULNAR

1. Simply assess pronation and supination.
2. Palpate the muscle barrier at the radial head.
3. During supination, the radial head glides anterior.
4. During pronation, the radial head glides posterior.
5. During supination and pronation there should be no medial or lateral motion of the radial head.
6. Palpate for medial and lateral motion of the radial head during supination and pronation.

POSITIONAL DIAGNOSIS–PROXIMAL RADIOULNAR

Supinated	The radial head is stuck supinated in anterior glide and cannot pronate with posterior glide.
Pronated	The radial head is stuck pronated in posterior glide and cannot supinate with anterior glide.

MOVEMENT BARRIER—PROXIMAL RADIOULNAR

Supinated: Passive pronation should not occur with lateral glide of radial head.

- Palpate muscle barrier of lateral glide of the radial head.

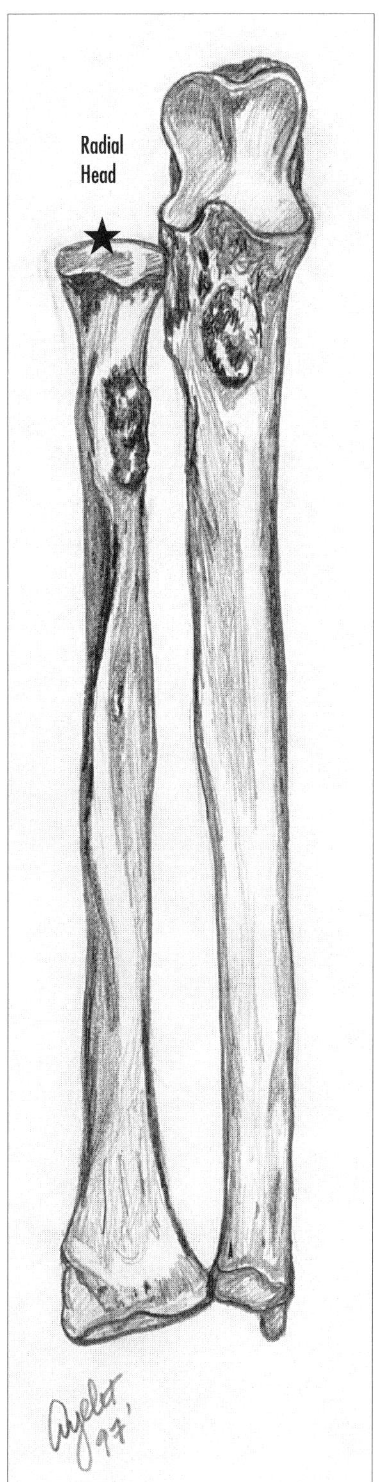

Figure 13. Palpate the radial head. The radial head glides anterior during supination. The radial head glides posterior during pronation. Lateral glide of the radial head should not occur during supination or pronation.

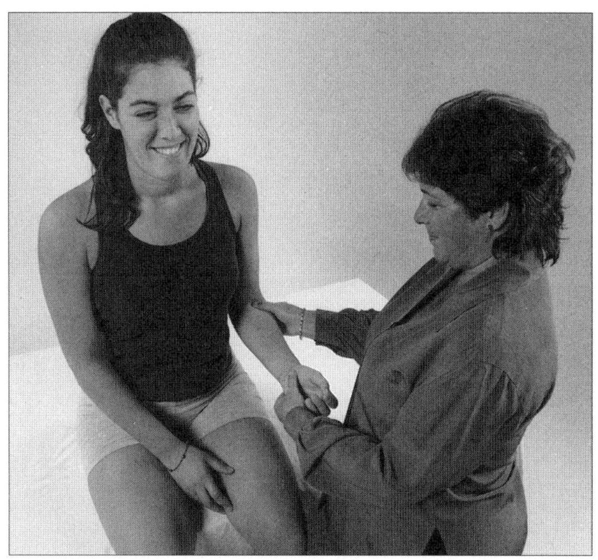

Treatment for supinated radioulnar joint. Palpate lateral movement of radial head for barrier.

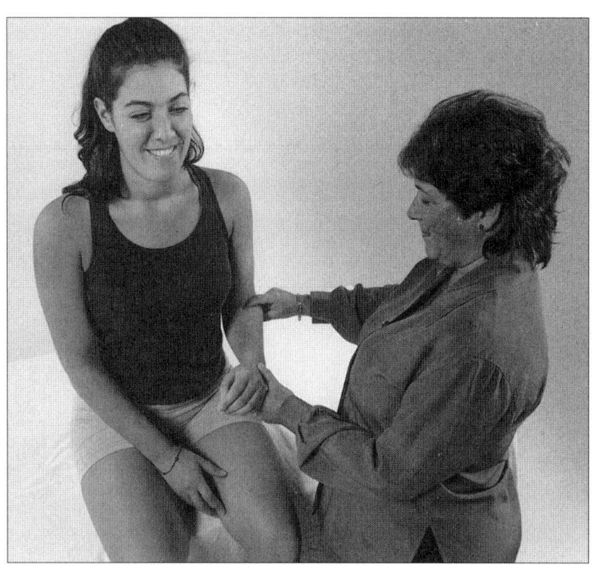

Treatment for pronated radioulnar joint. Palpate lateral movement of radial head for barrier.

Pronated: Passive supination should not occur with medial glide of radial head

- Palpate muscle barrier of medial glide of the radial head.

POSITION OF TREATMENT–PROXIMAL RADIOULNAR

Supine or sitting with elbow flexion at 90 degrees, shoulder in 0 degrees abduction, 0 degrees flexion, and 0 degrees rotation.

Supinated — The proximal radioulnar joint is stuck Supinated.

Movement barrier: Pronation.

Pronated — The proximal radioulnar joint is stuck Pronated.

Movement barrier: Supination.

TREATMENT–PROXIMAL RADIOULNAR

Supinated

1. Passively pronate the forearm, until the interbarrier zone. Palpate for lateral glide of the radial head.
2. Resist supination or pronation. Isometric resistance; 6 seconds resistance; 5 grams of force.
3. Relax.
4. Repetition: 3.
5. Reassess.

Pronated

1. Passively supinate the forearm, until the interbarrier zone. Palpate for lateral glide of the radial head.
2. Resist supination or pronation. Isometric resistance; 6 seconds resistance; 5 grams of force.
3. Relax.
4. Repetitions: 3.
5. Reassess.

The Radiohumeral Joint

The radiohumeral joint is the joint where elbow extension occurs. The humeroulnar joint is the joint where flexion occurs.

This radiohumeral joint gets stuck Flexed: The movement barrier is Extension. The radiohumeral joint cannot extend.

ASSESSMENT–RADIOHUMERAL

1. During elbow extension, which primarily occurs at the radiohumeral joint, there is anterior glide of the radial head.
2. During elbow extension with supination (after 0 degrees neutral through 90 degrees supination), there is anterior glide of the radial head.
3. During elbow extension with pronation (after 0 degrees neutral through 90 degrees pronation), there is anterior glide of the radial head with longitudinal distraction of the radial head (rather than posterior glide, which occurs with pronation in flexion).
4. Extension is considered 0 degrees.
5. Flexion is any elbow flexion after 0 degrees.
6. Therefore, during elbow extension from flexion, in supination and in neutral (0 degrees supination/pronation), the radial head is gliding anterior from a posterior glide position.
7. During elbow extension after 0 degrees, which is hyperextension, there is anterior glide of the radial head.
8. When supination is present, there is anterior glide of the humeral head. When pronation is present, there is a longitudinal distraction of the radial head.
9. In extension, there should be no medial or lateral glide at the radial head.

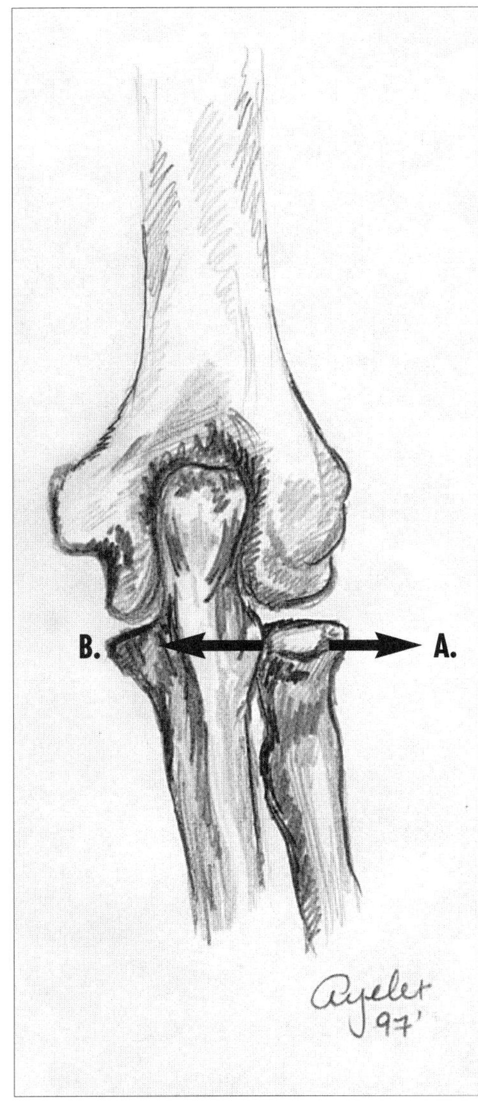

Figure 14. Palpate for **A.** medial and **B.** lateral motion of the radial head for the barrier.

POSITIONAL DIAGNOSIS–RADIOHUMERAL

Flexed, Pronated	Find in Extension: Stuck Flexed. During Extension, palpate lateral glide of the radial head: Stuck Pronated.
Flexed, Supinated	Find in Flexion: Stuck Extended. During Extension, palpate medial glide of the radial head: Stuck Supinated.

MOVEMENT BARRIER–RADIOHUMERAL

Palpate the muscle barrier at the radial head. There should be no medial or lateral movement of the radial head during extension. *Palpate for medial and lateral motion of the radial head in extension.*

Flexed, Pronated	The radiohumeral joint is stuck Flexed and Pronated. The elbow cannot Extend and Supinate. Movement barrier: Extension, Supination
Flexed, Supinated	The radiohumeral joint is stuck Flexed and Supinated. The elbow joint cannot Extend and Pronate. Movement barrier: Extension, Pronation

POSITION OF TREATMENT–RADIOHUMERAL

Flexed, Pronated	Positional diagnosis: Flexed, Pronated Movement barrier: Extension, Supination The position of treatment is the same as the movement barrier: Extension, Supination.
Flexed, Supinated	Positional diagnosis: Flexed, Supinated Movement barrier: Extension, Pronation The position of treatment is the same as the movement barrier: Extension, Pronation.

TREATMENT–RADIOHUMERAL

1. In supine or in sitting: shoulder joint at 0 degrees abduction, 0 degrees rotation, 0 degrees flexion.
   - Position forearm at 0 degrees supination/pronation.
   - Flex the elbow to 100 percent flexion.
   - Passively extend the elbow from 100 percent flexion.
2. Palpate the radial head for medial and lateral glide of the radial head.
   - If there occurs lateral glide of the radial head, the positional diagnosis is: Flexed, Pronated.
   - If there occurs medial glide of the radial head, the positional diagnosis is: Flexed, Supinated.
3. Extend to the interbarrier zone (before medial or lateral glide of the radial head).
4. Take into movement barrier of pronation or supination to interbarrier zone.
5. Isometric resistance: supination or pronation; 5 grams force; 6 seconds resistance.
6. Relax.
7. Progress to next interbarrier zone.
8. Repetitions: 3.
9. Reassess.

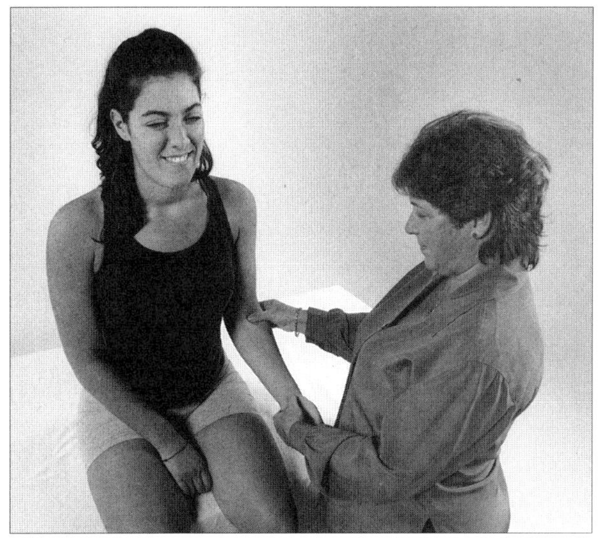

Treatment of flexed, pronated radiohumeral joint: extend the elbow from full flexion. Palpate for lateral glide of the radial head.

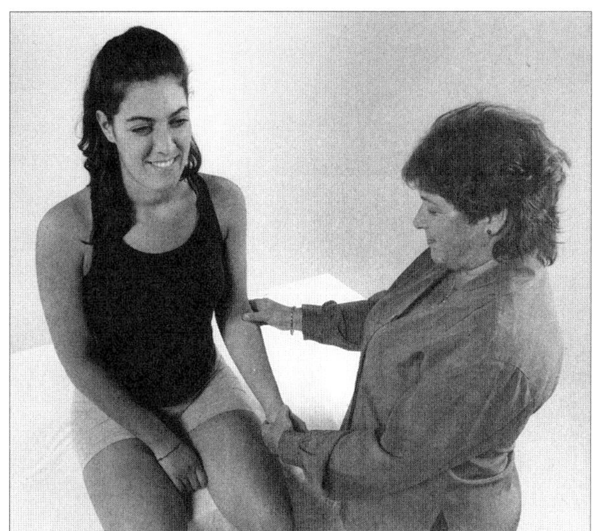

Treatment of flexed, supinated radiohumeral joint: extend the elbow from full flexion. Palpate for medial glide of the radial head.

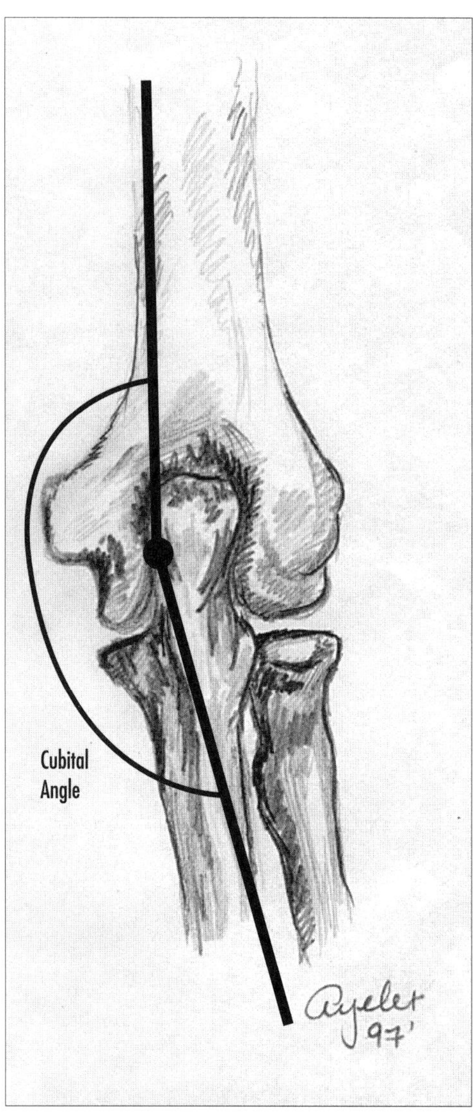

Figure 15. Palpate the barrier at the cubital angle. Any presentation of a cubital angle before 0 degrees (full extension) reflects humeroulnar joint dysfunction.

The Humeroulnar Joint

This joint is the primary flexion joint for the elbow. Therefore, there are extended dysfunctions that prevent flexion.

ASSESSMENT–HUMEROULNAR

Palpate the muscle barrier at the cubital angle. There should be no cubital angle until full extension. Full extension is 0 degrees flexion. At 0 degrees there is angulation with medial gap that occurs during the locking mechanisms only. *Also palpate medial and lateral glide of the radial head in flexion.*

POSITIONAL DIAGNOSIS–HUMEROULNAR

Extended, Supinated	Find in Flexion: Stuck Extended.
	During Flexion, palpate medial glide of the radial head: Stuck Supinated.
Extended, Pronated	Find in Flexion: Stuck Extended.
	During Flexion, palpate lateral glide of the radial head: Stuck Pronated.

MOVEMENT BARRIERS–HUMEROULNAR

Extended, Supinated — The humeroulnar joint is stuck Extended, Supinated.

The elbow cannot Flex and Pronate.

Movement barrier: Flexion, Pronation.

Extended, Pronated — The humeroulnar joint is stuck Extended, Pronated.

The elbow cannot Flex and Supinate.

Movement barrier: Flexion, Supination.

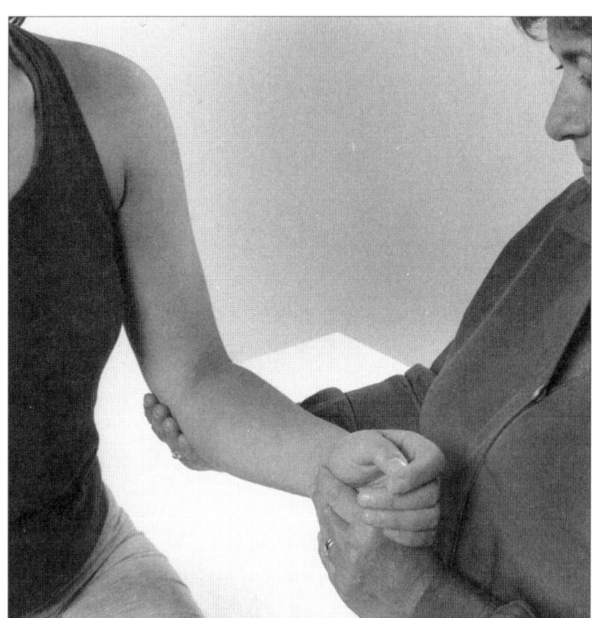

Treatment of extended, pronated humeroulnar joint. In neutral forearm, flex the elbow. The cubital angle will appear with a lateral glide of the proximal radial head.

POSITION OF TREATMENT–HUMEROULNAR

Extended, Supinated — Positional diagnosis: Extended, Supinated.

Movement barrier: Flexion and Pronation.

The position of treatment is the same as the movement barrier: Flexion and Pronation.

Extended, Pronated — Positional diagnosis: Extended, Pronated.

Movement barrier: Flexion and Supination.

The position of treatment is the same as the movement barrier: Flexion and Supination.

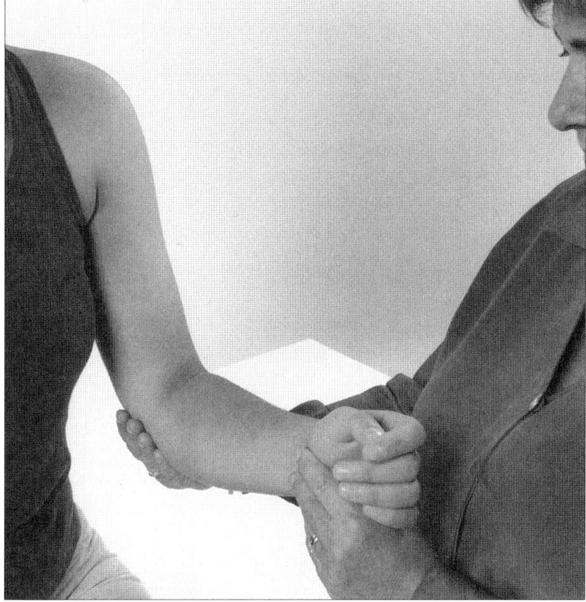

Treatment of extended, supinated humeroulnar joint. In neutral forearm, flex the elbow. The cubital angle will appear with a medial glide of the radial head.

TREATMENT–HUMEROULNAR

1. In supine or sitting:
   shoulder is at 0 degrees abduction,
   0 degrees rotation, 0 degrees flexion.
2. Position the forearm in 0 degrees pronation/supination.
3. Position the elbow joint in full extension.
4. Passively flex the elbow joint.
5. Palpate the muscle barrier at the cubital angle. As soon as the cubital angle increases, the barrier has been reached. Go to the interbarrier zone, immediately before the cubital angle starts to appear.
6. When the cubital angle appears with lateral glide of the proximal radial head, the positional diagnosis is: Extended, Pronated.
7. When the cubital angle appears with medial glide of the proximal radial head, the positional diagnosis is: Extended, Supinated.
8. Resistance: elbow flexion or extension; isometric; 6 seconds resistance; 5 grams force.
9. Relax.
10. Progress to the next interbarrier zone.
11. Repetitions: 3.
12. Reassess.

Wrist Joints

The radiocarpal joint(s) are the primary joint(s) of wrist extension.
The ulnarcarpal joint(s) are the primary joint(s) of wrist flexion.

The proximal carpal row joints in articulation with the distal carpal row joints are the primary joints for radial and ulnar deviation.

The radiocarpal joint(s) and the ulnarcarpal joint(s) are easy to attain excellent articular balance and good mobility with Muscle Energy and 'Beyond' Technique philosophy.

Direct accessory movements are as follows:

- During physiologic extension there is anterior glide of the proximal carpal row.
- During physiologic flexion there is posterior glide of the proximal carpal row.
- During physiologic radial deviation there is medial glide of the distal carpal row.
- During physiologic ulnar deviation there is lateral glide of the distal carpal row.

ASSESSMENT–WRIST JOINTS

1. The distal carpal row glides medial for radial deviation.
2. The distal carpal row glides lateral for ulnar deviation.
3. Palpate the movement barrier at the medial and lateral aspects of the distal carpal row. Flexion and extension of the wrist joint occur without ulnar and radial deviation.

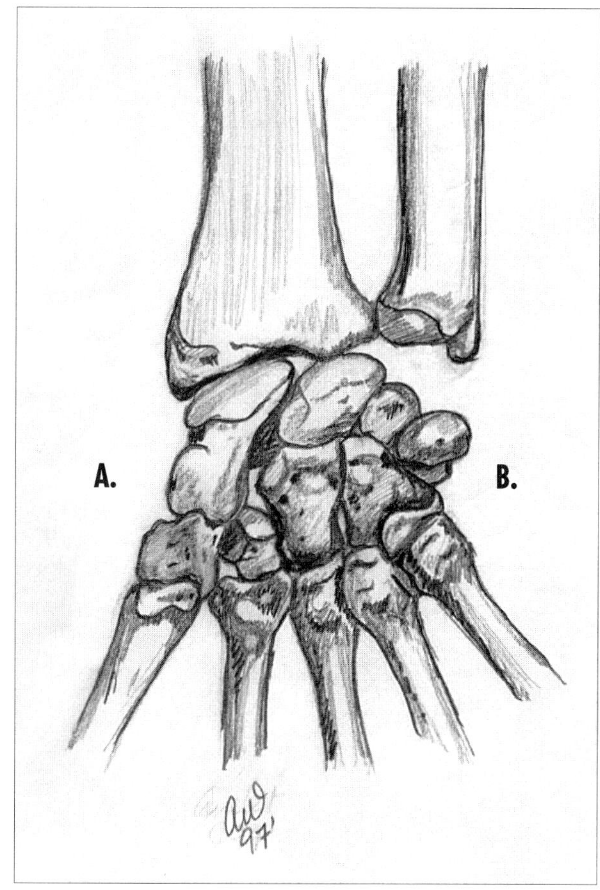

Figure 16. Palpate for wrist joint dysfunction at the distal carpal row. Ulnar and radial deviation manifest at the distal carpal row. **A.** The distal row glides medial for radial deviation. **B.** The distal row glides lateral for ulnar deviation.

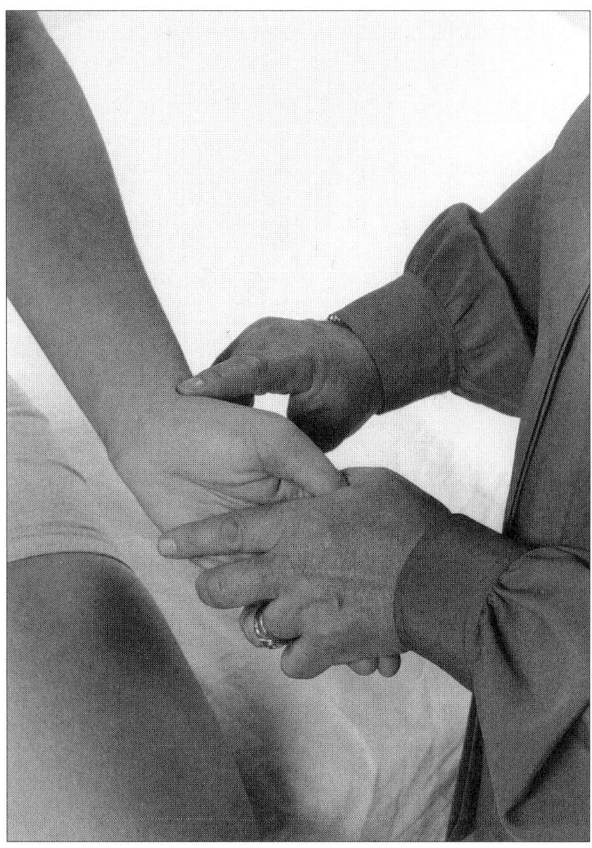

Treatment of flexed, ulnar deviated: extend the wrist. Palpate lateral glide of the distal carpal row. Resist any wrist movement.

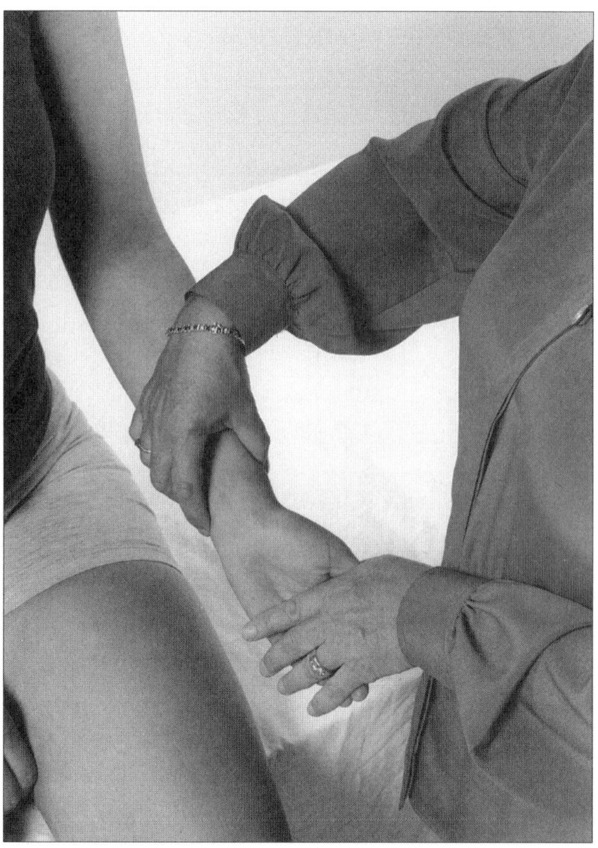

Treatment of flexed, radial deviated: extend the wrist. Palpate medial glide of the distal carpal row. Resist any wrist movement.

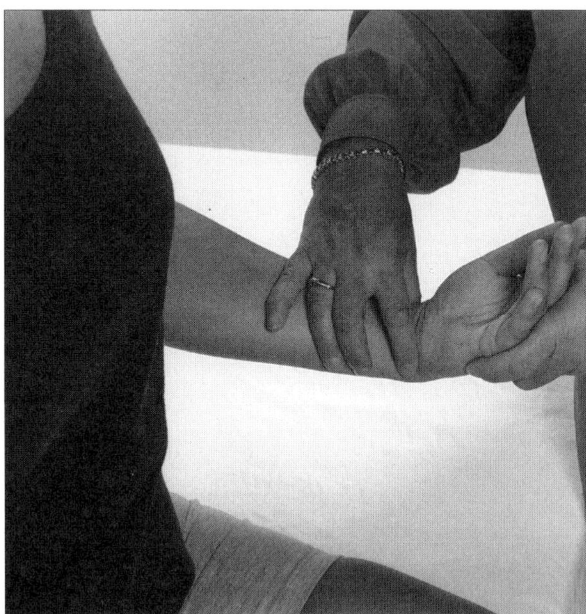

Treatment of extended, ulnar deviated: flex the wrist. Palpate lateral glide of the distal carpal row. Resist any wrist movement.

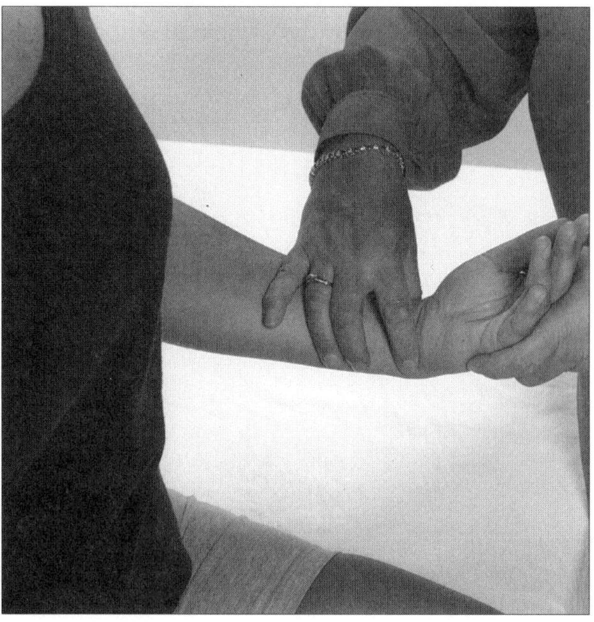

Treatment of extended, radial deviated: flex the wrist. Palpate medial glide of the distal carpal row. Resist any wrist movement.

POSITIONAL DIAGNOSIS–WRIST JOINTS

Flexed, Ulnar Deviated	Find in Extension: Stuck Flexed. During Extension, palpate lateral glide of distal carpal row: Stuck Ulnar Deviated.
Flexed, Radial Deviated	Find in Extension: Stuck Flexed. During Extension, palpate medial glide of distal carpal row: Stuck Radially Deviated.
Extended, Ulnar Deviated	Find in Flexion: Stuck Extended. During Flexion, palpate lateral glide of distal carpal row: Stuck Ulnar Deviated.
Extended, Radial Deviated	Find in Flexion: Stuck Extended. During Flexion, palpate medial glide of distal carpal row: Stuck Radially Deviated.

MOVEMENT BARRIER–WRIST JOINTS

Flexed, Ulnar Deviated	The wrist is stuck Flexed. The distal carpal row is stuck in lateral glide. Movement barrier: Extension and Radial Deviation.
Flexed, Radial Deviated	The wrist is stuck Flexed. The distal carpal row is stuck in medial glide. Movement barrier: Extension and Ulnar Deviation.
Extended, Ulnar Deviated	The wrist is stuck Extended. The distal carpal row is stuck in lateral glide. Movement barrier: Flexion and Radial Deviation.
Extended, Radial Deviated	The wrist is stuck Extended. The distal carpal row is stuck in medial glide. Movement barrier: Flexion and Ulnar Deviation.

POSITION OF TREATMENT–WRIST JOINTS

Flexed, Ulnar Deviated

Extend the wrist. Palpate lateral glide of the distal carpal row. Return to the interbarrier zone, just before lateral glide of the distal carpal row. Do radial deviation to the interbarrier zone. Resist any wrist movement. Isometric resistance; 5 grams of force; 6 seconds resistance. Relax. Progress to next interbarrier zone. Repeat 3 repetitions. Reassess.

Flexed, Radial Deviated

Extend the wrist. Palpate the medial glide of the distal carpal row. Return to the interbarrier zone, just before medial glide of the distal carpal row. Do ulnar deviation to the interbarrier zone. Resist any wrist movement. Isometric resistance; 5 grams of force; 6 seconds resistance. Relax. Progress to next interbarrier zone. Repeat 3 repetitions. Reassess.

Extended, Ulnar Deviated

Flex the wrist. Palpate lateral glide of the distal carpal row. Return to the interbarrier zone, just before lateral glide of the distal carpal row. Do radial deviation to the interbarrier zone. Resist any wrist movement. Isometric resistance; 5 grams of force; 6 seconds resistance. Relax. Progress to next interbarrier zone. Repeat 3 repetitions. Reassess.

Extended, Radial Deviated

Flex the wrist. Palpate the medial glide of the distal carpal row. Return to the interbarrier zone, just before medial glide of the distal carpal row. Do ulnar deviation to the interbarrier zone. Resist any wrist movement. Isometric resistance; 5 grams of force; 6 seconds resistance. Relax. Progress to next interbarrier zone. Repeat 3 repetitions. Reassess.

TREATMENT–WRIST JOINTS

1. In supine or sitting: position the shoulder in 0 degrees abduction, 0 degrees rotation, 0 degrees flexion.
2. Position the elbow joint at 90 degrees flexion.
3. Position the forearm in 0 degrees supination/pronation.
4. Begin from 0 degrees neutral wrist flexion/extension.
5. Palpate lateral aspects of the distal carpal row to assess muscle barriers.

CHAPTER 6

SYNERGIC PATTERN IMPRINT AND SYNERGIC PATTERN RELEASE

A MODEL FOR TREATMENT OF PROTECTIVE MUSCLE SPASM

Using a Synergic Pattern Release (SPR) for elimination and reduction of protective muscle spasm, joint mobility and articular balance is typically restored. This Synergic Pattern Release was discovered by (Weiselfish) Giammatteo while adapting Jones' Strain and Counterstrain Technique for the neurologic patient. The author found that typical patterns of muscles in spasm repeatedly presented themselves in the clients with neurologic deficits. These patterns were then tested on populations of clients who did not manifest patho-neurologic disorders. These patterns (synergic patterns) were present in the non-neurologic population as well, consistently. The author hypothesizes that "imprints" of these synergic patterns are DNA characteristics. She calls this manifestation: Synergic Pattern Imprint.

What are Synergic Patterns? This term has been present in patho-neurology literature for many decades. Persons with spasticity present typical postural deviations which are the result of certain muscles in a state of sustained involuntary contraction. Typically the same muscles are always in severe muscle spasm, contributing to similar postural appearances.

Synergic Pattern Imprint of the Lower Extremity

The typical synergic pattern of the lower extremity consists of the following postures:

- Flexed lumbosacral junction
- Elevated pelvis
- Retracted pelvis
- Flexed hip joint
- Internally rotated hip joint
- Adducted hip joint
- Flexed knee joint (although with closed head injury clients an extended knee presentation is not uncommon)
- Plantar flexed ankle joint
- Supinated varus foot is common

The soft tissue and joint articular balance problems within this manifestation of the lower extremity include the following:

- Approximated femoral head
- Caudal femoral head
- Internal rotated femoral head
- Lateral glide of the proximal tibial articular surface
- Superior patella
- External rotation of the gastrocnemius belly
- Anterior distal tibia on talus
- Flexed calcaneus

Synergic Pattern Imprint of the Upper Extremity

The typical synergic pattern of the upper extremity includes the following postures:

- Forward head and neck with flexed C7 on T1
- Elevated shoulder girdle
- Protracted shoulder girdle
- Flexed shoulder joint
- Adducted shoulder joint
- Internally rotated shoulder joint
- Flexed elbow joint
- Increased cubital angle
- Pronated forearm
- Flexed wrist joint (although the closed head injury client often presents an extended wrist)
- Ulnar deviated wrist
- Flexed fingers
- Flexed thumb
- Adducted thumb

The soft tissue and joint articular balance problems within this manifestation of the upper extremity include the following:

- Elevated first rib at the costovertebral joint
- Caudal humeral head
- Anterior humeral head
- Approximated humeral head
- Anterior proximal radial head
- Medial gap of the ulna
- Posterior distal radial head
- Anterior distal ulna head
- Anterior proximal carpal row
- Approximated first proximal metacarpal head
- Anterior first proximal metacarpal head

The Synergic Pattern Imprint is present in all persons. When a person receives a neurologic insult, the typical inhibited pattern of hypertonicity will be disinhibited. All of the suppressed hyperactivity will surface. The result is the spastic synergic pattern which is typical of every hemiplegic patient. The person who sustains a closed head injury will present a similar pattern of spasticity, with slight variations.

The author noted during many years of research that the patterns of hypertonicity in the mild neurologic patient were almost exactly like the patterns of hypertonicity in the severe chronic pain person. This stimulated her to observe more closely the relative impressions of tone and postures presented by all persons, of different ages, different diagnoses. It became evident that the presentation of the typical synergic pattern of hypertonicity is present in all persons, but inhibited until there is a release of this inhibition. All persons can benefit from treatment addressed towards release of the synergic pattern of hypertonicity, known as Synergic Pattern Release (see Chapters 9, 10, and 11).

CHAPTER 7

A HYPOTHETICAL MODEL

EXPLAINING THE DECREASE OF HYPERTONICITY WITH MANUAL THERAPY

This chapter presents the (Weiselfish) Giammatteo model to support all results with manual therapy.

The musculofascialskeletal system receives most of the efferent outflow from the central nervous system; the largest portion of this efferent discharge exits the spinal cord via the ventral roots to the muscles. The musculofascialskeletal systems are also the source of much of the widespread, continuous, and variable sensory input to the CNS. This sensory feedback relayed from receptors in myofascial, visceral, articular components, and others, enters the spinal cord via the dorsal roots. This sensory reporting is routed to many centers throughout the central nervous system, including the cerebral cortex, the cerebellum, the brain stem, and the autonomic nervous system. This sensory input from the musculofascialskeletal body is extensive, intensive, and continuous, and is a dominant influence on the central nervous system.

The Premise

Disturbances in the sensory afferent input from the neuromusculoskeletal systems, whether diffuse or local, affect motor functions and other functions. This premise is a core concept, clinically significant for hypertonicity (protective muscle spasm and spasticity), the Facilitated Segment, and Structural Rehabilitation.

In 1947, Denslow stated a hypothesis which explained this concept:

> (An) osteopathic lesion represents a facilitated segment of the spinal cord maintained in that state by impulses of *endogenous origin* entering the corresponding dorsal root. All structures receiving efferent nerve fibers from that segment are, therefore, potentially exposed to excessive excitation or inhibition.

The site of this *endogenous origin* is the proprioceptors, especially the muscle spindles. They are sensitive to musculofascialskeletal stresses. They are non-adapting receptors, sustaining streams of impulses for as long as they are mechanically stimulated. Their influence is specific to the muscles acting on the affected joints, which are innervated by corresponding spinal segments.

The Myotatic Reflex Arc

The Myotatic Reflex Arc (also known as the stretch reflex arc, the monosynaptic reflex arc, and the gamma motor neuron loop) has long been considered as the basis of muscle tone. The components of this reflex arc include: the muscle fiber, which has the ability to contract and to relax and elongate; the muscle spindle, the proprioceptor, which is responsive to length and velocity stretch; the gamma neuron, which innervates the muscle spindle; the afferent neuron, which transcribes the information regarding stretch to the spinal cord; and the alpha motor neuron, which transcribes the impulse from the spinal cord to the muscle fiber, eliciting a muscle contraction.

The Muscle

The muscle is the focus of dysfunctional movement, when considering the hypertonicity of protective muscle spasm and spasticity. The muscle is active, self-energized, independent in motion and capable of developing great, widely variable, and rapidly changing forces. Other tissues are passively moved, immobilized, pushed, pulled, compressed, and altered in shape by those forces of muscular origin. Muscles *produce motion* by their contraction, but those same contractile forces also *oppose motion*. Contracting muscle absorbs momentum, and regulates, resists, retards, and arrests movement. Irving Korr states that this energy-absorbing function of skeletal muscle is as important to the control of motion as its energy-imparting function. But the same cellular mechanisms are involved in these functions.

Joint mobility, range of motion, and ease of initiation of active motion are results of healthy muscle function. Limited capacity of muscles often appears to be the major impediment to mobility of a dysfunctional joint. Korr states that muscular resistance is not based on inextensibility, as with connective tissues, but on changes in the degree of activation and deactivation of the contractile tissue. The hypothetical cause for a muscle to increase or decrease its contraction and braking power is variations in impulse flow along the motor axons, the alpha neurons, which innervate the muscle. This neuronal impulse traffic varies with changing levels of excitation within the anterior horn cells, which change according to varying afferent input.

Proprioceptors

The muscle spindle, the proprioceptor within the muscle fibers which responds to stretch, is a basic component of the myotatic reflex arc, and has been implicated as a basic component of protective muscle spasm, and of spasticity. The proprioceptors are the sensory end organs that signal physical changes in musculofascialskeletal tissues. The three main categories of proprioceptors are sensitive to joint position and motion, to tendon tension, and to muscle length.

The *joint receptors* are located in joint capsules and ligaments; they report joint motion and position. The Ruffini endings in the capsules report direction, velocity of motion, and position very accurately. These joint receptors do not appear to have significant influence on motor activity via the stretch reflex arc, although this premise is presently under investigation.

The *Golgi tendon receptors* are located in tendons close to the musculotendinous junction. A pull on the tendon causes discharge of impulses into the spinal cord via afferent fibers. This pull is usually exerted by active contraction of the muscle. The tendon endings are responsive to changes in force, not in length. When the muscle contracts against a load, or fixed object, or against the contraction of antagonistic muscles as in spasticity and protective muscle spasm, the discharge of the tendon endings is in proportion to the tension that is developed. The afferent input from the Golgi tendon varies with the tension exerted by the muscle on the tendon, regardless of the muscle length. The discharges of the tendon endings enter the spinal cord by dorsal root fibers, where they excite *inhibitory* interneurons that synapse with motor neurons controlling the same muscle. The effect of their discharge is inhibitory; it tends to oppose the further development of tension by the muscle.

The Muscle Spindle

The *muscle spindles* are complex. Each spindle has two kinds of sensory endings with different reflex influences, each with its own motor innervation. Spindles are scattered throughout each muscle, the quantity varying according to the function of the muscle and the delicacy of its control. The greater the spindle density, the finer the control. The complex anatomy and physiology of the muscle spindles is well documented in the literature.

Spindles are within the muscle itself, surrounded by muscle fibers, arranged in parallel with them and attached to them at both ends. Stretching the muscle causes stretch of the spindle; shortening of the muscle slackens the spindle. Each spindle, enclosed in a connective tissue sheath, about 3 mm long, has several thin muscle fibers. These are the *intrafusal fibers.* The larger and more powerful *extrafusal fibers* comprise the bulk of the muscle. The intrafusal fibers are attached to the sheath at each end. *The intrafusal muscle fibers are innervated by gamma motor neuron fibers* originating in the ventral horn, passing through the ventral root. *The alpha motor neurons supply innervation to the extrafusal muscle fibers.*

The sensory endings of the spindle are in close relation to the central, nucleated, noncontractile portion of the intrafusal fibers. This sensory ending, called the *primary ending*, is wound around the intrafusal fibers, described as the *annulospiral ending. Secondary flower-spray endings* occur on either side of the primary ending and are connected to thinner myelinated axons. Both are sensitive to stretch of the central portion of the spindle.

There is a static and a dynamic response to stretch by the muscle: static is proportional to muscle length; dynamic is proportional to the rate of change in muscle length. The intrafusal muscle fiber is relatively elastic: the 1A afferent endings, which innervate the primary nerve endings, end here. Therefore, the 1A fiber has a dynamic and a static response to stretch. The group II afferent fibers, which innervate the secondary endings, end on the small nuclear chain fibers. This is at the area of the myofibril striations of the intrafusal fibers: a less elastic, stiffer area. Therefore there is only a static response to stretch which is proportional to muscle length. Since these fibers have no dynamic response, they will not carry central nervous system feedback regarding the velocity of the stretch.

The primary endings, or *annulospiral endings, respond to change in muscle length.* When the muscle is stretched beyond its resting length, the spindle is stretched, causing the primary and secondary endings to fire at increased frequencies in proportion to the degree of stretch. Shortening of the muscle, whether by its own contraction or by passive approximation of its attachments, slows the discharge proportionately, and may even silence it.

The spindle, an essential feedback mechanism by which the muscle is controlled, continually reports back to the central nervous system. The feedback from the primary endings of each spindle is conveyed by dorsal root fiber directly, that is, monosynaptically, to the alpha motor neurons of the same muscle. This afferent discharge of the spindle results in excitation of the alpha motor neurons of the same muscle. How does this occur? *When a muscle is stretched, it is reflexively stimulated by its spindles to contract*, and thereby resists stretching. This protective reflex response is at the spinal cord level of the same spinal segment. *The protective shortening of the muscle decreases the afferent discharge,* and thus reduces the excitation of the alpha motor neurons, *causing relaxation and lengthening of the muscle.*

The muscle spindle causes the muscle to resist change in length in either direction. The spindle is the sensory component of the stretch, reflex arc, or myotatic reflex arc. It is important in the maintenance of posture.

The intrafusal muscle fibers influence spindle discharge. Their ends are anchored, and contraction of these intrafusal fibers stretches the middle portion in which the sensory endings are situated, increasing their discharge. *The effect of intrafusal contraction on the sensory endings is indistinguishable from the effect produced by stretch of the extrafusal fibers.* The two effects are cumulative. At any lengthening of the muscle, intrafusal contraction would increase the spindle discharge; stretch of the muscle while the intrafusal fibers are contracted produces a more intense spindle discharge than when the intrafusal fibers are at rest or less contracted.

The Gamma Neuron

The gamma neuron, a component of the myotatic reflex arc (or gamma motor neuron loop), innervates the muscle spindle, is affected by dysfunction within the neuromusculoskeletal system, and is controlled by the brain and supraspinal neurons. The function of the gamma neurons is to control contraction of the intrafusal fibers, the frequency of the spindle discharge at a given muscle length, and the sensitivity or change in that frequency per millimeter change in length. The higher the gamma activity, the larger the spindle response; the higher the spindle discharge at a given muscle length, the shorter the length of muscle at which a given impulse frequency is generated. *This explains the threshold to stretch of the spindle.*

The gamma neurons, also known as *fusimotor* neurons, are small in size and their axons are thin. Fusimotor innervation by the gamma fibers comprises one-third of the ventral root outflow from the spinal cord. Alpha-to-gamma and extrafusal-to-intrafusal relationships regulate the activity of skeletal muscles. *The higher the spindle discharge, the greater the reflex contraction of the muscle.* What that muscle contraction accomplishes depends on the other forces acting on the joints crossed by that muscle. Generally, the greater the contraction, the more the muscle shortens and moves the joint, and the more it resists being stretched in the opposite direction.

Gamma Bias

Normal resting conditions of gamma activity maintain a tonic afferent discharge from the spindle. This is the *gamma bias.* This maintains the alpha motor neurons in a moderately facilitated state and the muscles in low-grade tonic contraction at their resting lengths. Thus, people are not flaccid and hypotonic, but maintain some muscle tone. Gamma activity may be turned up or down. The higher the gamma activity, because of its influence on the excitatory spindle discharge, the more forceful the muscle's contraction and the greater its resistance to being lengthened. During high gamma activity, or *gamma gain,* the spindle may elicit contraction when the muscle is already shorter than its resting length. If the increased gamma gain is sustained, the muscle contraction is maintained. This is muscle spasm.

The sensory endings of the spindle are stimulated by mechanical distortion, whether caused by contraction of the intrafusal fibers or by stretch of the main muscle, or both. The spindle in effect reports length *relative* to that of the intrafusal fibers. The greater the disparity in length, the greater the discharge and the greater the contraction of the muscle. Increase in intrafusal-extrafusal disparity increases the afferent discharge, which results in a contractile response of the extrafusal fibers, which in turn tends to reduce the disparity and to silence the spindle. *The greater the gamma activity, the more the muscle must shorten before the spindle is turned back down to resting discharge and normal gamma bias. The central nervous system can elicit and precisely control gamma bias.*

There is always some activity around this myotatic reflex arc. There is a certain *gamma bias: a certain level of activity along the gamma neuron which results in a resting threshold to stretch of the muscle spindle, controlled by the central nervous system.* Evidently, the gamma neuron is inhibited by supraspinal structures. When there is a cortical lesion, the suppressor areas of the brain which inhibit the gamma neuron are damaged. The inhibition process via the medial reticular formation is affected. An increased level of activity within the myotatic reflex arc occurs because of the resultant increase in gamma bias. Gamma bias is no longer normal, due to disinhibition of the central nervous system. The result is spasticity, which is hypertonicity, plus other characteristics of the syndrome of spasticity. The gamma gain and the hyperactivity of the myotatic reflex arc result in the hypertonicity of protective muscle spasm and spasticity.

The Afferent Neuron

Whenever the muscle spindle is stimulated, via stretch stimulus, that information passes along the afferent neuron into the posterior horn of the spinal cord of that spinal segment. Some of this sensory input is distributed throughout the central nervous system. Much of the sensory input passes as discharge along the same afferent neuron to the anterior horn of that same spinal segment. In the ventral horn, this discharge passes across the synapse to the neuron of the alpha motor nerve, and passes along the length of the alpha motor neuron axon to the muscle fiber. When the muscle fiber receives the impulse, it contracts and shortens.

Neuromusculoskeletal Dysfunction and the Hyperactive Myotatic Reflex Arc

This hypothetical model expands on Denslow's and Korr's hypothesis of the osteopathic lesion, in order to provide a model which explains the results of manual therapy for treatment of neuromusculoskeletal dysfunction. These results include increased resting muscle length, increased joint mobility, and increased ranges of motion.

A Hypothetical Model

Envision a cross section of the spinal cord at the level of C5. The embryologic segment of C5 spinal cord innervates certain tissues and structures. Among these tissues and structures are: the supraspinatus muscle, the deltoid muscle, the infraspinatus muscle, the subscapularis muscle, the biceps muscle (C5, 6), and more. When there is dysfunction in one or more of the tissues and structures which are innervated by the C5 embryologic segment, there is resultant increase in gamma gain and protective muscle spasm of the musculature innervated by that same C5 segment.

Neuromusculoskeletal Dysfunction Causes Afferent Gain; Afferent Gain Causes Alpha Gain

When a person has a supraspinatus tendinitis, the brain is apprized of this status. The person perceives pain at the shoulder. The pain is generic: The person does not know that the pain is the result of a supraspinatus dysfunction. *The afferent neuron, bringing the sensory information about this dysfunction to the spinal cord, will pass this information as excessive and high frequency discharge.* This is similar to the excessive and high frequency discharge of gamma gain, but it is "afferent gain." The afferent neuron from the supraspinatus muscle and tendon will pass the sensory information along the afferent neuron as increased afferent gain, which enters the spinal cord via the dorsal roots and posterior horn of C5 spinal segment.

This excessive and high frequency discharge is distributed throughout the central nervous system: cortex, brain stem, up one or more spinal segments, down one or more spinal segments, across to the opposite side of the spinal cord, and more. Some of this excessive and high frequency discharge is also passed along the afferent neuron to the anterior horn. At the ventral horn, the excessive and high frequency discharge passes across the synapse and affects the alpha motor neuron which innervates the supraspinatus muscle. This same excessive and high frequency discharge passes along the length of the alpha motor neuron which innervates the supraspinatus muscle.

This excessive and high frequency discharge, passing down the length of the alpha motor neuron to the muscle fiber, is *alpha gain*, or the increase in discharge and activity of the alpha motor neuron. When an impulse reaches the muscle fiber, the muscle fiber contracts and shortens. If excessive and too frequent discharge passes along the alpha motor neuron, the muscle fiber will go into a state of contraction which is sustained by the continuous volley of impulses. The muscle fiber, the supraspinatus, can no longer voluntarily relax and elongate. This is the model of *protective muscle spasm* of the supraspinatus which results from a supraspinatus tendinitis dysfunction.

If there is a supraspinatus tendinitis, the supraspinatus muscle will go into a state of protective muscle spasm, contracted and shortened, incapable of attaining full resting length due to an inability to relax and elongate. The supraspinatus crosses the glenohumeral joint. The joint surfaces will become approximated, resulting in joint hypomobility and limitations in ranges of motion.

Gamma Gain: Increased Sensitivity of the Muscle Spindle and Decreased Threshold to Stretch

The excessive and high frequency discharge which is passed into the alpha motor neuron in the anterior horn is also passed into the gamma motor neuron. Alpha and gamma signals are linked and coordinated in the spinal segment. The gamma motor neuron passes this excessive and high frequency discharge down to the muscle spindle. The muscle spindle is now hyperinnervated. Therefore, the sensitivity of the spindle to stretch is increased; the threshold of the muscle spindle to stretch will be decreased. The spindle will be "hyperactivated," and will react to smaller stretch, and lower velocity of stretch, than before the supraspinatus tendinitis was present. There is a facilitation of the myotatic reflex arc: *The stretch reflex arc is hyperactive.* This phenomenon is called a *facilitated segment.*

The Facilitated Segment and Efferent Gain of Alpha and Gamma Neurons

Increased efferent gain is characteristic of the facilitated segment. The alpha motor neurons which innervate the supraspinatus muscle fibers are not the only neurons to exit from the anterior horn of C5 embryologic segment. The other alpha neurons, for example, those which innervate the subscapularis, infraspinatus, deltoid, and biceps (C5, 6), can also pass the excessive and high frequency discharge accumulating in the ventral horn, as the condition of the supraspinatus tendinitis becomes more severe and more chronic. This excessive and high frequency discharge in the anterior horn, when sufficient to influence the other neurons, will pass along those other alpha motor neurons innervated by the same C5 spinal segment. *Thus there is a potential and tendency for protective muscle spasm of all the muscles innervated by that same C5 embryologic segment which innervates the supraspinatus. This situation becomes exacerbated as the tendinitis becomes more severe and more chronic.*

The gamma neurons, which innervate the intrafusal muscle fibers of the muscle spindles of all the muscles innervated by this same C5 embryologic segment, can also pass this excessive and high frequency discharge, as the dysfunction becomes more severe and more chronic. *As a result, the sensitivity of these spindles to stretch is increased, and the threshold to stretch of all the muscle spindles innervated by this spinal segment is decreased.* The potential for protective muscle spasm and dysfunction is exacerbated. All these muscles cross the glenohumeral joint, therefore the approximation of the humeral head in the glenoid fossa, the joint hypomobility, the disturbance of articular balance, and the limitations in ranges of motion are exacerbated.

Somatovisceral Reflex Arcs

Neurons exiting the spinal cord innervate more than muscle spindles and muscle fibers. They also provide innervation of viscera via the autonomic nervous system. For example, L1 innervates the cecum. If a patient with a history of an appendectomy has scarring within the lower right abdominal cavity, this information will be passed as sensory feedback via the afferent neurons to the central nervous system. Afferent neurons, passing this information as excessive and high frequency discharge, enter the spinal cord via the posterior horn of L1. From here the sensory information is distributed throughout the central nervous system. Some of the information is also relayed to the anterior horn of this same L1 embryologic segment. All the alpha motor neurons which are innervated by L1 embryologic segments can potentially pass this excessive and high frequency discharge, which is accumulating in the L1 anterior horn, and can pass this hyperactivity along the alpha motor neurons, which would result in protective muscle spasm of the muscle fibers innervated by that same L1 segment. Also, all the muscle spindles innervated by the gamma neurons from this L1 segment which could potentially pass the excessive and high frequency discharge will be affected, so that the threshold to stretch of all these muscle spindles would be decreased. This facilitated segment at L1, the result of dysfunctional tissue surrounding the cecum, may cause somatic dysfunction of the pelvis and hip joint region because of the sustained contraction of the muscles crossing those joints.

Manual Therapy to Decrease Hypertonicity

If all of the neuromusculoskeletal fascial dysfunction is treated, there will be a decrease and/or elimination of afferent gain, and thereby a decrease in the hyperactivity of the myotatic reflex arc. The efferent gain will be reduced. The muscle tone will be normal. When treatment of neuromusculoskeletalfascial dysfunction is not sufficient to decrease the hypertonicity, Jones' Strain and Counterstrain Technique will decrease and/or eliminate the muscle spasm.

CHAPTER 8

THE MUSCLE BARRIER

If the muscle spindle is hyperinnervated due to gamma gain, the threshold to stretch of that muscle spindle is lowered. In a healthy muscle, during passive movements, the muscle spindles should not be stimulated throughout the normal range of motion. There should be a reasonable stretch on each muscle before the spindle, the stretch receptor, is activated. In passive movement, there should not be any assistance, or any resistance, by the muscle fibers. But if the muscle spindle is hyperinnervated, during passive stretch the muscle spindle will react and a stretch reflex will be activated. Afferent impulses from the spindle will go into the dorsal root of the posterior horn, and many of these impulses will continue along to the anterior horn. The afferent neuron will synapse with the alpha motor neuron in the anterior horn. The impulses will be transcribed along the neuron, and the muscle fiber will contract.

The muscle barrier is the threshold of the muscle spindle of the stretched muscle to stimulus of stretch.

A passive movement was performed. The threshold to stretch of the muscle spindle was reached. A stretch reflex arc was activated. The muscle contracted. The movement was no longer passive. There was now a muscle contraction which resisted further passive movement. *At the first moment of muscle contraction, the muscle barrier was met. The first moment of muscle contraction was the moment that passive movement was first resisted by that muscle.*

The interbarrier zone is a few degrees of motion before the muscle barrier.

Example: Biceps Muscle Barrier

Elbow extension is performed passively. Initially, the movement is passive: There is no assistance by the elbow extensors, and no *resistance by the biceps*. But the muscle barrier is finally reached. The degree of elbow extension is reached which finally exerts too much of a stretch on the muscle spindle of at least one biceps muscle fiber. The threshold to stretch of the muscle spindle of this first biceps muscle fiber is met. The muscle spindle begins to fire. The impulses are transcribed along the afferent neuron, into the spinal cord via the posterior horn, and over to the anterior horn. The impulses cross the synapse, and continue along the axon of the alpha motor neuron to the biceps muscle fiber. That biceps muscle fiber contracts. The elbow extension is now no longer passive. There is resistance from the muscle contraction of the biceps muscle fiber.

The barrier is the place in the passive range of motion when the first muscle fiber contracts and resists the passive movement.

Energy Expenditure Due to the Resistance of a Muscle in Protective Muscle Spasm

Observation

Test assisted active prone knee bending. Observe all postural deviations of the leg. Maintain the neck and shoulder girdle at neutral. Do not allow the forearm, wrist, hand or fingers to deviate from neutral/midline during movement. The therapist may need to passively maintain neutral of distal arm during movement. Ask the patient to *actively extend the elbow*. Observe the difficulty in initiating and continuing the movement when the distal arm and shoulder girdle are forced to maintain neutral/midline posture. Movement requires good articular balance.

Application of the Muscle Barrier Concept

Hypothesis

Hypertonicity (protective muscle spasm) in a muscle will inhibit range of motion in the opposite direction.

- Example: Hamstrings (hip extensors) spasm inhibits straight leg raise (hip flexion).
- Example: Hamstrings (knee flexors) spasm inhibits knee extension.
- Example: Right hip adductors spasm inhibits right hip abduction and right lumbar side bending.
- Example: Right scalenes spasm inhibits left cervical side bending.

Hypothesis

Hypertonicity in a muscle will inhibit range of motion in the opposite direction from muscle origin and from muscle insertion.

- Example: Iliacus (hip flexors) spasm inhibits hip extension and lumbar extension.
- Example: Spasm of the upper left rib depressor muscles will inhibit left shoulder abduction.

Analysis and Interpretation of Postural Dysfunction

Static Postural Dysfunction

The body part deviates *towards* the protective muscle spasm and spasticity due to contracted and shortened muscle fibers. The *range of motion* will be *limited in the opposite direction.*

Dynamic Postural Dysfunction

Consider the muscle in spasm as the agonist. The range of motion is limited in the opposite direction, opposite the agonist's direction of primary movement, because of the resistance by the agonist. For example, if the biceps (the agonist) are in spasm, then elbow extension is limited because the biceps will resist the pull of the triceps (the antagonist).

CHAPTER 9

TREATMENT OF HYPERTONICITY

FOR SYNERGIC PATTERN RELEASE WITH STRAIN AND COUNTERSTRAIN TECHNIQUE

Thank you, Dr. Jones.

This segment of this book is dedicated to Lawrence Jones, D.O. His contribution to manual therapy and health care will be recognized by all who use his approach, Strain and Counterstrain Technique.

The author has modified somewhat Jones' original approach in order to optimize effects for the neurologic, pediatric, geriatric and chronic pain patient to a "corrective kinesiologic" approach. This approach was founded on Jones' Strain and Counterstrain Technique.

Sharon (Weiselfish) Giammatteo, Ph.D., P.T.

Direct and Indirect Techniques

Manual therapy is comprised of direct and indirect techniques. Direct techniques load, or bind, the tissues and structures. The tissue is moved towards a barrier, on one or more planes. The direction of movement is towards the least mobile, most restricted, most limited. At the barrier a technique is performed, and the result is a change of the position of the barrier, closer to the normal range of motion. Muscle Energy and 'Beyond' Technique is a direct technique. For example, if there is an elbow flexion contracture, with contracted and shortened biceps, and a limitation of elbow extension, the elbow would be moved into extension, on three planes. At the 3-planar interbarrier zone, an isometric resistance is performed. The result is increased range of extension motion. Mobilization and manipulation are also direct techniques.

Indirect techniques unload, or ease, the tissues and structures. The tissue is moved away from the barrier, on one or more planes. The direction of movement is towards the most mobile, least restricted, least limited. The distortion is, thereby, exacerbated. The problem is exaggerated. The result would be a "Release" phenomenon, when the soft tissues "let go" allowing increased range of motion past the original barrier. For example, if there is an elbow flexion contracture, with contracted and shortened biceps, and a limitation of elbow extension, the elbow would be moved into flexion with two other planes added. After 90 seconds, a "Release" phenomenon would occur, resulting in decreased hypertonicity and increased elongation of the biceps, and increased range of extension motion. Strain and Counterstrain is an indirect technique.

Treatment of Muscle Fiber Hypertonicity with Strain and Counterstrain Techniques

Strain and Counterstrain Technique was developed by Lawrence Jones, D.O. This technique is a positional technique which results in decrease or arrest of inappropriate proprioceptor activity of the muscle spindle. The result of this technique is a relaxation and elongation of the muscle fiber, which permits improved articular balance, for increased joint mobility and range of motion.

Dr. Jones has isolated tender points throughout the trunk, extremities, and cranium of the body which reflect: (1) a muscle in spasm, or (2) a compressed joint or suture. When neuromusculoskeletal dysfunction is present, with protective muscle spasm and/or joint dysfunction with approximating articular surfaces, the correlating tender point is painful on palpation. When the body part is positioned appropriately, the pain of the tender point diminishes or disappears immediately. Maintaining the body part in the correct position, which shuts off the painful tender point, will result in a correction of the dysfunction after 90 seconds duration.

As the muscle fibers relax and elongate during the treatment technique, there is a decrease in the exaggerated push/pull function of the muscle. The muscle decreases its forceful pull on the bone. There is a resulting increase in joint mobility while there is a repositioning of the articular surfaces. The patient often senses the movement, because the kinesthetic receptors in the joints, for example the Ruffini, receive the sensory input of movement and change of position in space during the technique. It is important that the therapist does not change the position of the body part during the technique.

As long as the patient is experiencing any movement or tissue tension change, or the therapist is palpating movement or tissue tension change, the body position should be maintained. Only when the patient and the therapist no longer experience any tissue changes or movement, can the body part be slowly and gently returned to a neutral position.

Every tender point discovered by Dr. Jones is effective. The techniques outlined in this course and these handouts will be very effective in reducing the protective muscle spasm typical in upper quadrant dysfunction. The learner is advised to learn more Strain and Counterstrain Techniques once a comfort level with this technique has been achieved.

As mentioned above, all the Strain and Counterstrain Techniques are effective. The therapist can focus on an area of postural asymmetry, or hypomobility, and perform the tender points in those areas.

The criteria for implementing the techniques are always the same:

1. Position the body part as close as possible with the instructions to shut off the painful trigger.
2. Maintain the position for 90 seconds.
3. After the 90 seconds, do not move the position if the patient or therapist is still experiencing any tissue tension changes or movement. (This is a De-Facilitated Fascial Release.)
4. When all tissue tension changes have stopped and there is no movement experienced, the body part should be gently and slowly returned to a neutral position.

Corrective Kinesiology: Model of Strain and Counterstrain Technique

Objective: Corrective Kinesiology

Elimination of hypertonicity allows elongation of the muscle fibers to their normal resting length, which diminishes the pathologic tension of the muscle on the bone, which results in normalization of joint biomechanics.

Hypothetical Objective with Strain and Counterstrain Technique

Goal

Shorten the muscle fiber of the agonist (hypertonic muscle) and strain the Golgi tendon of the antagonist: to decrease the gamma gain to the spindle of the agonist; and to decrease the hyperactivity of the myotatic reflex arc of the agonist.

Objective

Exaggerate the postural deviation: Go indirectly into the direction of pull of the already contracted and shortened muscle tissue.

Result

Elongation of the muscle fiber without stretching, and increased joint mobility and range of motion.

Evaluation Process for Hypertonicity of the Muscle Fiber with Strain and Counterstrain Technique

An effective and efficient technique to reduce and arrest inappropriate proprioceptor activity of the muscle spindle, to diminish and eliminate the hyperactivity within the reflex arc, is Strain and Counterstrain Technique, developed by Lawrence Jones, D.O. The result of comprehensively eliminating hyperactivity within the facilitated segment is an elongation of the muscle fiber to its true resting length. When the muscle fiber is healthy and elongated, it does not exert abnormal and pathologic tension on the bone, in either direction of pull: insertion towards origin, or origin towards insertion. There is no pathologic force from this muscle fiber causing a shift in bony position and a change in the neutral position of the articular surfaces of that bone. The muscle fiber is not contributing to an imbalance of the articular surface. Therefore, the result achieved with elimination of protective muscle spasm is a normalization of the positions of the articular surfaces of the joints, with increased joint mobility and increased range of motion.

The increased physiologic range of motion is the result of:

- *elongation of the muscle fiber,*
- *increased joint mobility due to improved articular balance.*

Strain and Counterstrain Tender Points

Dr. Jones discovered painful Tender Points throughout the body. Each Tender Point is reflective of a muscle in protective muscle spasm, or a joint or suture which is compressed. He developed an evaluation process which systematically discovers the position of these Tender Points. The Tender Points discovered in the patient are documented. After the evaluation, all the severe Tender Points in the body are treated. Discovering a painful Tender Point, followed by elimination of the painful Tender Point with treatment, reflects a dysfunction successfully treated. A diagnosis is made. Typically, concurrent with the elimination of the painful point after treatment is a decrease in subjective pain, and an increase in range of motion.

The author recommends that the practitioner use the Mechanical Corrective Kinesiologic Approach. This approach to using Strain and Counterstrain Techniques recommends against the use of Tender Points. Placing pressure on a Tender Point in a client with protective muscle spasm will cause facilitation of the sympathetic nervous system and an increase in the hyperfacilitation of that muscle that is already in protective muscle spasm.

A Kinesiologic Approach for Evaluation of Hypertonicity

The postural evaluation described in this course and these handouts indicates those muscles in shortened and contracted conditions. Postural dysfunction reflects the hypertonicity of the muscles in that region. The therapist can evaluate static posture and dynamic movement to discover which hypertonic and contracted musculature is contributing to the postural dysfunction. A kinesiologic approach is possible. *For example, if the shoulder girdle is protracted and there is a limitation of horizontal abduction, the pectoralis minor can be treated as the hypertonic muscle contributing to the protracted shoulder girdle. The Tender Point technique for the pectoralis minor is the depressed second rib.*

*The following Strain and Counterstrain Techniques are all adapted from the research and work of Dr. Lawrence Jones. Wherever there is a **Synergic Pattern Release** this technique is part of a protocol to release the Synergic Pattern Imprint.*

CHAPTER 10

TREATMENT OF LOWER QUADRANT HYPERTONICITY

FOR SYNERGIC PATTERN RELEASE WITH STRAIN AND COUNTERSTRAIN TECHNIQUE

Iliacus

Pelvic Dysfunction

EVALUATE

Limitation of Motion: Hip extension and lumbar extension.

TENDER POINT

1 inch medial and half inch caudal to ASIS. Deep in iliac fossa.

TREATMENT

- Supine.
- Bilateral hip flexion to 100 degrees.
- Bilateral knee flexion to 130 degrees.
- External rotation of both hips (knees separated and ankles crossed).
- Bring both knees to the ipsilateral side of the Tender Point to 10 degrees, while maintaining bilateral external rotation.
- **Synergic Pattern Release**

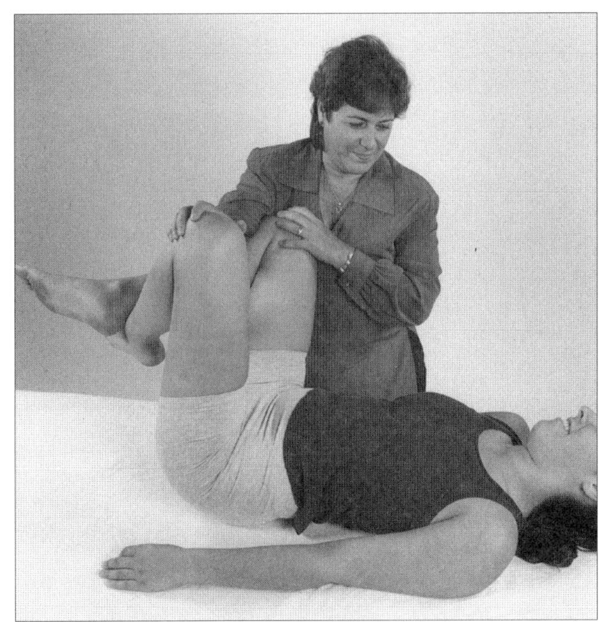

INTEGRATIVE MANUAL THERAPY

The iliacus is a powerful flexor of the hip, and flexes the lumbar and lumbosacral spine. Hypertonicity of the iliacus is common. This muscle compromises the vasculature of the inguinal canal, contributing to claudications and cramps of lower extremity musculature. Often the recurrences of joint dysfunction of the pelvic joints are secondary to iliacus spasm.

All Tender Points and techniques adapted from Jones' Strain and Counterstrain.

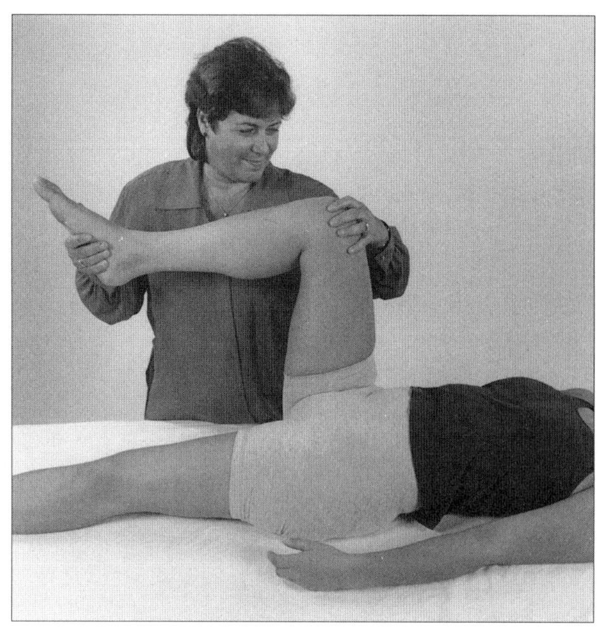

Medial Hamstrings

Pelvic Dysfunction

EVALUATE

Limitation of Motion: Hip flexion and lumbar flexion.

TENDER POINT

Just superior to the knee joint line on the medial border (possibly slightly posterior). On the attachment of the medial hamstrings to the posteromedial surface of the tibia.

TREATMENT

- Supine.
- Hip flexion to 90 degrees on the ipsilateral side.
- Knee flexion to 100 degrees on the ipsilateral side.
- Forceful external rotation of the ipsilateral tibia on the femur (2 to 5 pounds force).
- **Synergic Pattern Release**

INTEGRATIVE MANUAL THERAPY

The hamstrings are among the most often injured muscles. Often the injuries which are commonplace are secondary to pre-existing hamstrings spasm. This technique would be a valuable tool for all athletes, and can be taught to school team players to use on each other before and after games and heavy workouts, in order to reduce injury. The hamstrings spasm can directly cause meniscus torque, resulting in tendency of injury. The hamstrings are commonly cause for knee pain, gait deviations, and pressure of the vasculature in the popliteal fossa.

Adductor

Pelvic Dysfunction

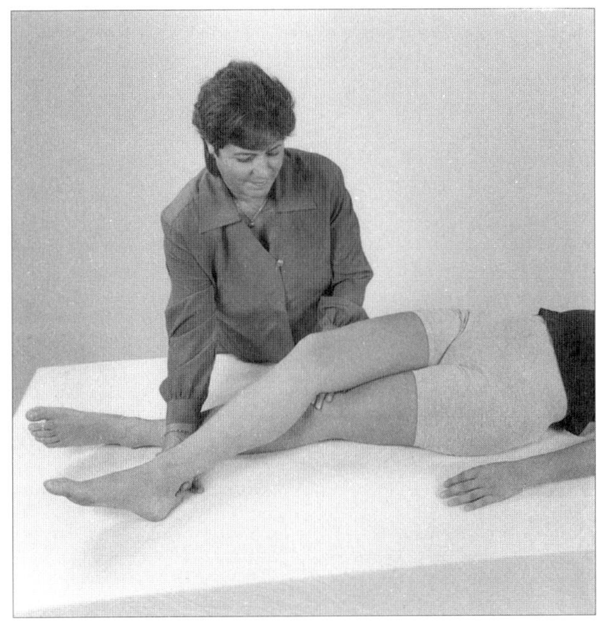

EVALUATE

Limitation of Motion: Hip abduction and ipsilateral lumbar side bending.

TENDER POINT

On the adductor tendon near the origin on the pubic bone.

TREATMENT

- Supine.
- Slight ipsilateral hip flexion. (Cross the treated leg over the opposite leg.)
- Adduction with overpressure.
- **Synergic Pattern Release**

INTEGRATIVE MANUAL THERAPY

Adductor muscle spasm is similar to tensions of the hamstrings in the torsion effects which result at the knee joint. There are multiple groin and hip joint problems which are caused by this muscle when it is in a state of contraction. The compression and caudal displacement of the femoral head, which is common in hip joint dysfunction, is mostly the result of adductor spasm.

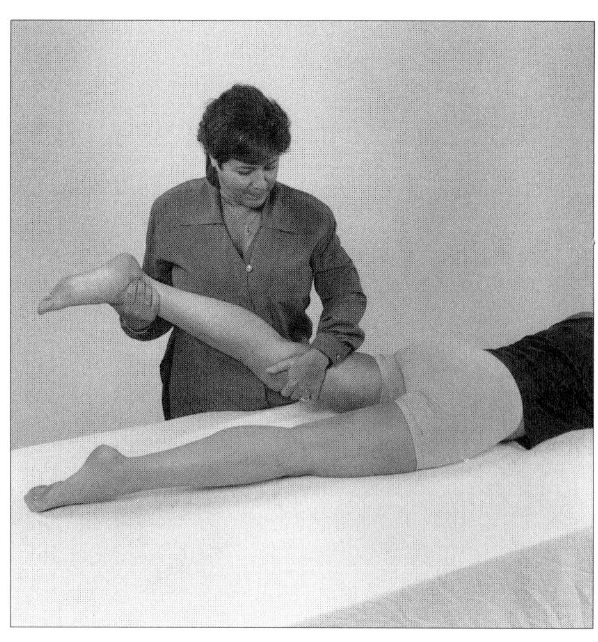

Gluteus Medius

Pelvis Dysfunction

EVALUATE

Limitation of Motion: Hip abduction and lumbar side bending to contralateral side.

TENDER POINT

Midaxillary line, 1 cm below the iliac crest.

TREATMENT

- Prone.
- Hip extension to 10 degrees on the ipsilateral side.
- Hip abduction to 10 degrees on the ipsilateral side.
- Hip internal rotation with overpressure.

Piriformis

Sacral Dysfunction

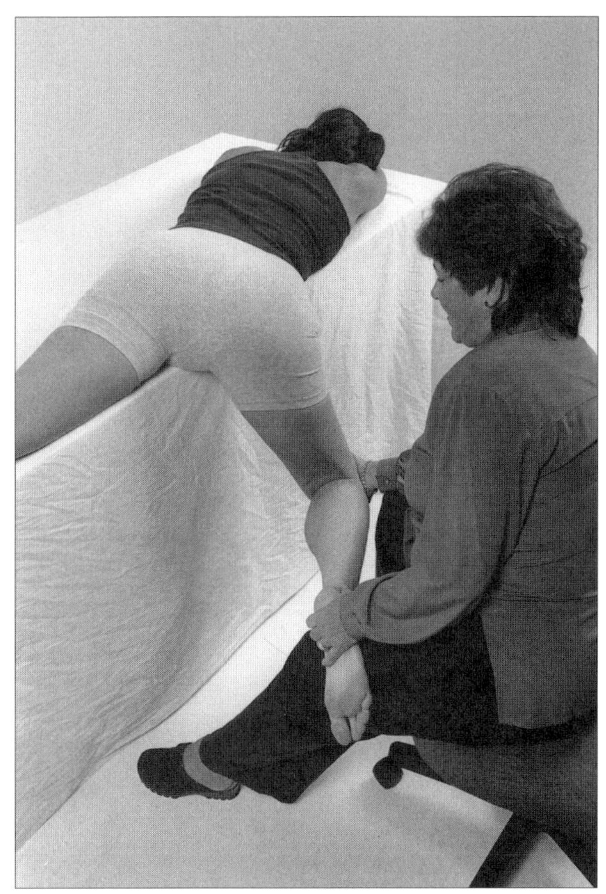

EVALUATE

Limitation of Motion: Hip internal rotation.

TENDER POINT

Find sacroiliac joint line; from a point at the middle of the joint line, make a line to the greater trochanter; in the middle of this line is the trigger.

TREATMENT

- Prone.
- Ipsilateral leg off the bed.
- Hip flexion to 120 degrees on the ipsilateral side.
- Knee flexion to 90 degrees on the ipsilateral side.
- Hip external rotation to 20 degrees on the ipsilateral side. (To effect rotation through the hip and pelvis.)
- Hip abduction to 10 degrees to the ipsilateral side.
- **Synergic Pattern Release**

INTEGRATIVE MANUAL THERAPY

The piriformis is a major external rotator of the hip. More significant is the function of torsion during ambulation. When the right heel strikes, the right piriformis contracts, and the sacrum is pulled into a left sacral torsion on a left oblique axis, required for stance phase. As the right foot goes from toe off towards swing phase, the tension of the piriformis subsides. An interesting characteristic of the piriformis muscle: There are multiple variations in muscle structure. The piriformis might be triangle shaped; it might be split, bifid. The piriformis originates from the anterior surface of the sacrum, and may receive fibers from any of the following places: the iliolumbar ligament, the sacrotuberous ligament, and more. In the majority of cadavers dissected, the sciatic nerve lies underneath the piriformis fibers. Often, this nerve runs between the fibers of a bifid piriformis. Rarely does the sciatic nerve lie on top of the piriformis. This is significant as a cause of pain and disability.

Whenever there is sacroiliac joint dysfunction, the piriformis muscle is in spasm. When the piriformis is in spasm, the muscle will contract and shorten and compress the tissue underneath it and between its fibers. Piriformis syndrome is the compromise of the sciatic nerve compressed underneath the muscle secondary to hypertonicity of that muscle.

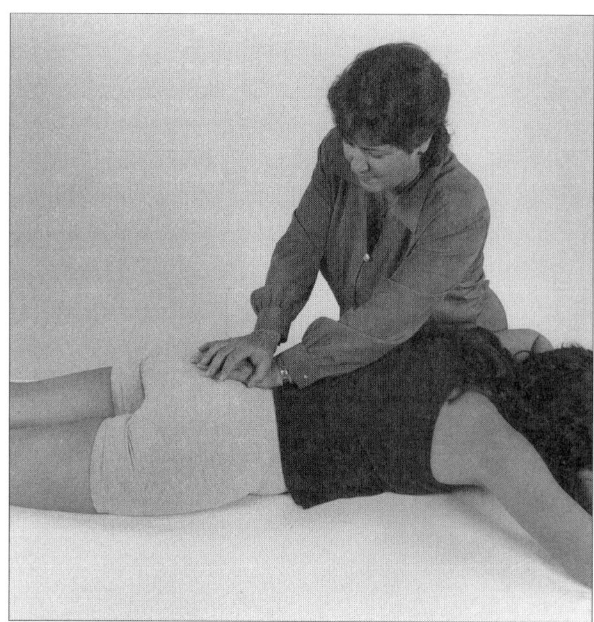

Treatment of the sacrum with Jones' Strain and Counterstrain Technique. (Tender Points #1, 2, 3)

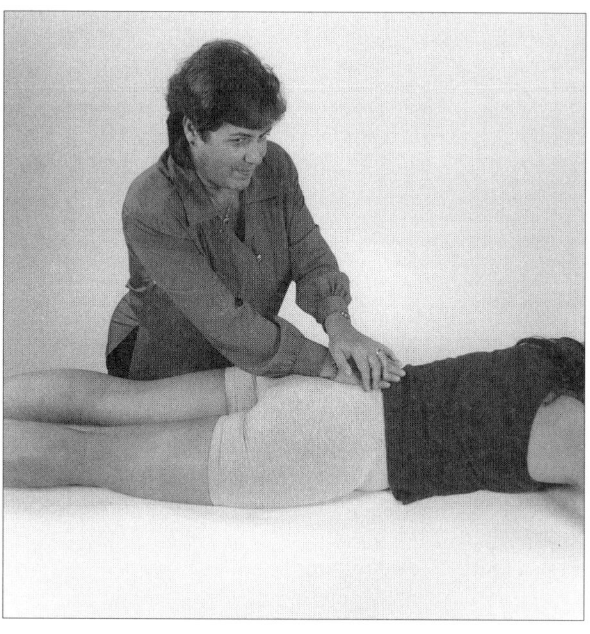

Treatment of the sacrum with Jones' Strain and Counterstrain Technique. (Tender Points #4, 5)

Treatment of Sacrum

Treatment of the sacrum with Jones' Strain and Counterstrain Technique is extremely effective. Note the location of the seven (7) sacral Tender Points. Press for 90 seconds on each Tender Point in the direction described below (1 through 5). The client is prone. Press hard enough for a response; not hard enough for a reaction!

TENDER POINTS

PS 1 (right & left)	1.5 cm medial to the inferior aspect of the posterior superior iliac spine.
PS 2	Midline on the sacrum between the first and second spinous tubercles.
PS 3	Midline on the sacrum between the second and third spinous tubercles.
PS 4	Midline on sacrum just superior to the sacral hiatus.
PS 5 (right & left)	1 cm medial and 1 cm superior to the inferior lateral angles bilaterally.

DIRECTION OF PRESSURE

Direction of pressure will be at the Tender Points listed above.

- PS 1: Posterior to anterior pressure (right and left).
- PS 2: Anteroinferior pressure (about 45 degrees angle).
- PS 3: Anteroinferior pressure (about 30 degrees angle).
- PS 4: Anterosuperior pressure (about 45 degrees angle).
- PS 5: Posterior to anterior pressure (right and left).

Anterior First Lumbar

Thoracolumbar and Lumbosacral Mobility

Restore reciprocal movement to the Lumbosacral Junction. L5/S1 is the seat of 3-planar reciprocal movement for gait ((Weiselfish) Giammatteo). Reciprocal movement is required for normal gait.

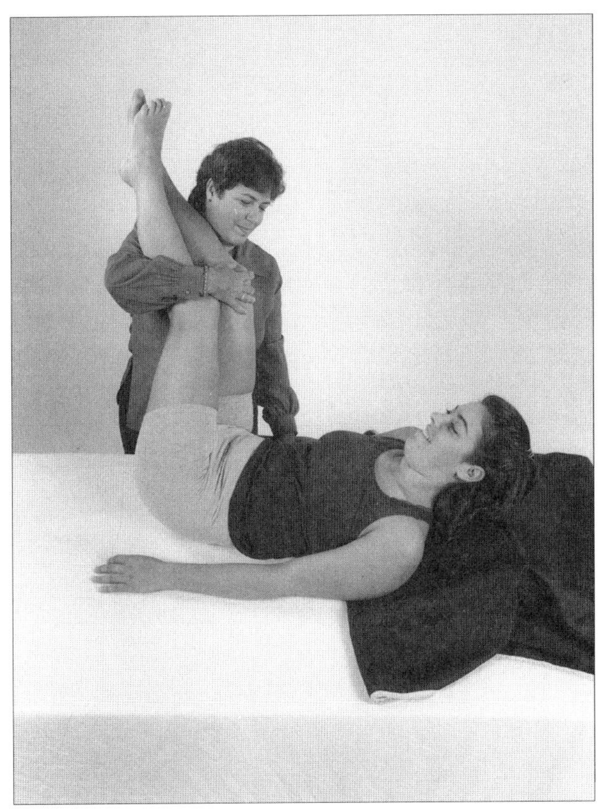

EVALUATE

Limitation of Motion: Lumbar extension and thoracolumbar mobility (segmental movement).

TENDER POINT

Push on medial aspect of ASIS, 3/4 inch deep.

TREATMENT

- Supine.
- Raise patient's head.
- Hip flexion to 120 degrees on the ipsilateral side.
- Knee flexion to 20 degrees on the ipsilateral side.
- Flex lumbar spine up the kinetic chain to L1.
- Rotate the knees 30 degrees to the ipsilateral side of the Tender Point, to attain about 5 degrees of trunk sidebend and about 40 degrees of trunk rotation.
- **Synergic Pattern Release**

INTEGRATIVE MANUAL THERAPY

There is a common dysfunction of the thoracolumbar junction: anterior shears of T12 and L1. This causes diaphragm spasm and is also a common compression source of L1 nerve root, resulting in hip joint pain. Anterior First Lumbar Strain and Counterstrain Technique can reduce the anterior shear of L1. In a similar manner, the Anterior T12 Strain and Counterstrain Technique can reduce the anterior and lateral shear of T12.

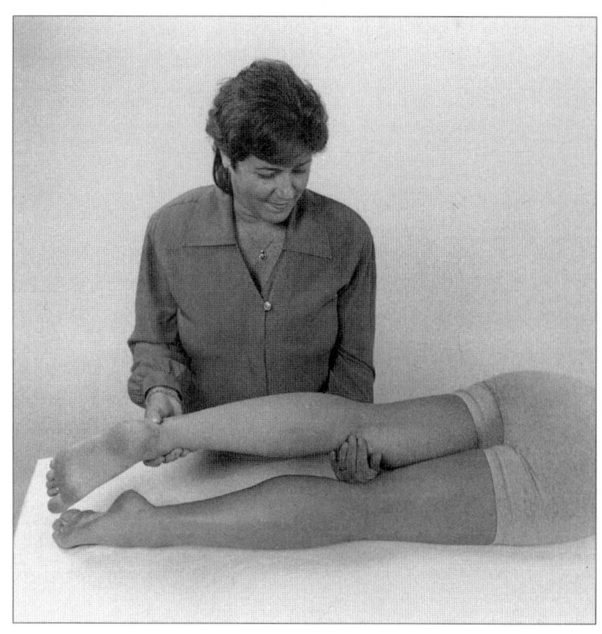

Posterior Fifth Lumbar Upper Pole

Thoracolumbar and Lumbosacral Mobility

EVALUATE

Limitation of Motion: Lumbosacral lumbar flexion (segmental movement).

TENDER POINT

Superior medial surface of PSIS.

TREATMENT

- Prone.
- Hip extension to 10 degrees on the ipsilateral side.
- Slight hip adduction (about 5 degrees) on the ipsilateral side.
- Slight hip external rotation (about 5 degrees) on the ipsilateral side.
- **Synergic Pattern Release**

INTEGRATIVE MANUAL THERAPY

This technique is valuable to decompress the lumbosacral junction. Prior to myofascial release or cranial therapy to open the fascial restrictions affecting L5/S1, this technique can be used.

Quadratus Lumborum: Anterior T12

Thoracolumbar and Lumbosacral Mobility

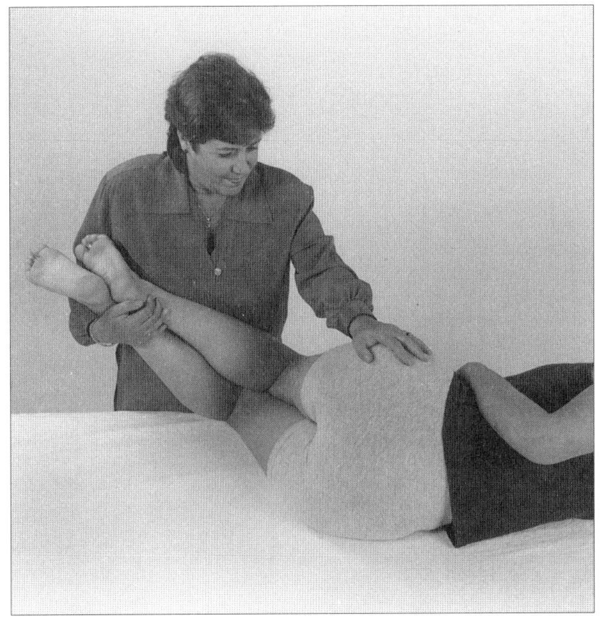

EVALUATE

Limitation of Motion: Lumbar side bending to opposite side.

TENDER POINT

Superior inner iliac crest (on the bone) in midaxillary line.

TREATMENT

- Side lying with the Tender Point side elevated. (Lie the client on the contralateral side.)
- Bilateral hip flexion to 45 degrees.
- Bilateral knee flexion to 90 degrees.
- Elevate the feet towards the ceiling to attain ipsilateral side bending of the trunk.
- **Synergic Pattern Release**

INTEGRATIVE MANUAL THERAPY

This technique is one of the most valuable contributions by Jones. The quadratus lumborum originates at the iliac crest, and inserts on the twelfth rib. When the quadratus lumborum is in spasm, it pulls the twelfth rib in an anterior and caudal direction. This is typical after major iliosacral joint dysfunction, such as an upslip or a downslip of the ilium. The result of a quadratus lumborum spasm: diaphragm spasm, anterior and lateral shears of T12, compression of the aorta or esophagus secondary to the dysfunction of the lower rib cage, and more.

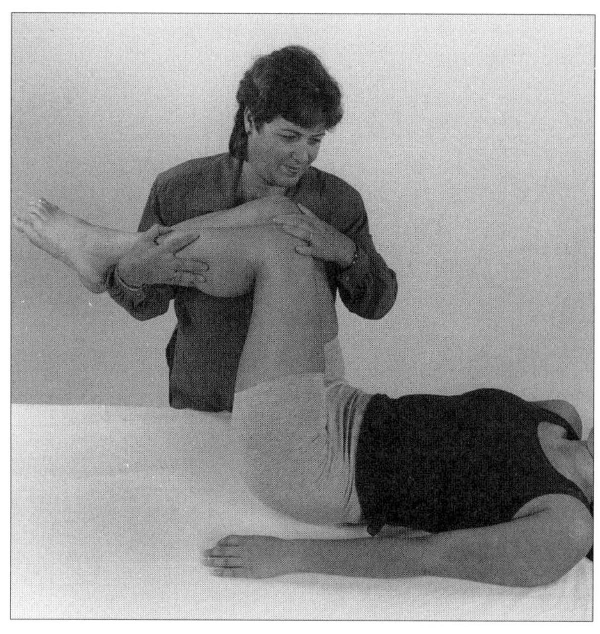

Anterior Fifth Lumbar

Thoracolumbar and Lumbosacral Mobility

EVALUATE

Limitation of Motion: Lumbosacral and lumbar extension.

TENDER POINT

Anterior surface of the pubic bone about 1.5 cm lateral to the pubic symphysis.

TREATMENT

- Supine.
- Bilateral hip flexion to 90 degrees.
- Bilateral knee flexion to 90 degrees.
- Move the knees 10 degrees to the ipsilateral side of the Tender Point, to attain the amount of trunk side bending and rotation required.
- **Synergic Pattern Release**

INTEGRATIVE MANUAL THERAPY

This is excellent first aid for lumbar strains. When the flexors of L5 are in spasm, they maintain L5 flexed, rotated and side bent. If the right flexor muscles of L5 are in spasm, the L5 will be flexed, rotated right and side bent right. The hydrostatic pressure on the disc will be affected. The disc will protrude posterior because of the flexed position; the disc will protrude to the left because L5 is stuck side bent to the right; there will be an increase in the intradiscal pressure directly proportionate to the angle rotation of L5. When this technique is performed, there is an elimination of the spasm, L5 is no longer maintained in a flexed, rotated and side bent position, the hydrostatic pressure on the disc is normalized, and the protruding disc will spontaneously be reduced.

Quadriceps (Patellar Tendon)

Knee Dysfunction

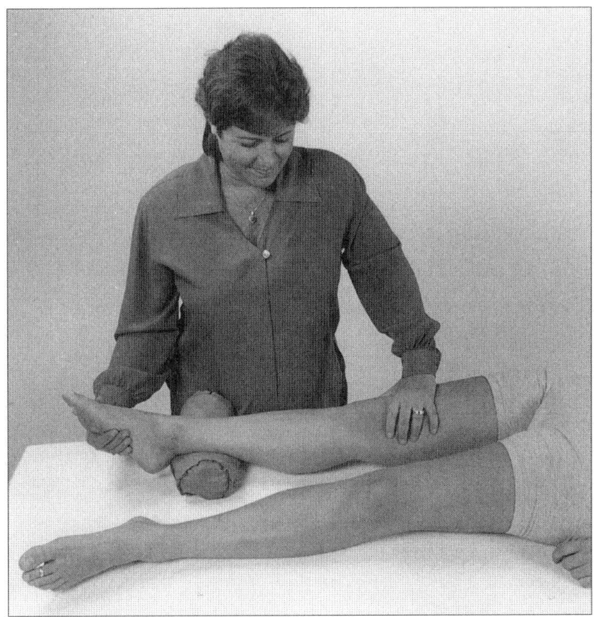

EVALUATE

Knee Flexion.

TENDER POINT

Medial portion of patellar tendon or tibial tubercle.

TREATMENT

- Supine.
- Place towel roll under the ipsilateral ankle.
- Slight inversion of the ipsilateral foot.
- Apply anterior to posterior pressure on femur, applied proximal to the ipsilateral knee, 5 to 10 pounds force.
- **Synergic Pattern Release**

INTEGRATIVE MANUAL THERAPY

The quadriceps spasm is often caused from a loss of dorsiflexion. When a person stands or walks without ten degrees of dorsiflexion, extensor forces are transcribed up the leg, and the quadriceps will go into a state of hypertonicity. It is important to restore dorsiflexion for healthy quadriceps tone. If the quadriceps is contracted, the patella will be compressed against the femur: a common cause of chondromalasia. Patella alta will result, and patella tracking will be affected by quadriceps spasm. Multiple problems may be alleviated with this technique.

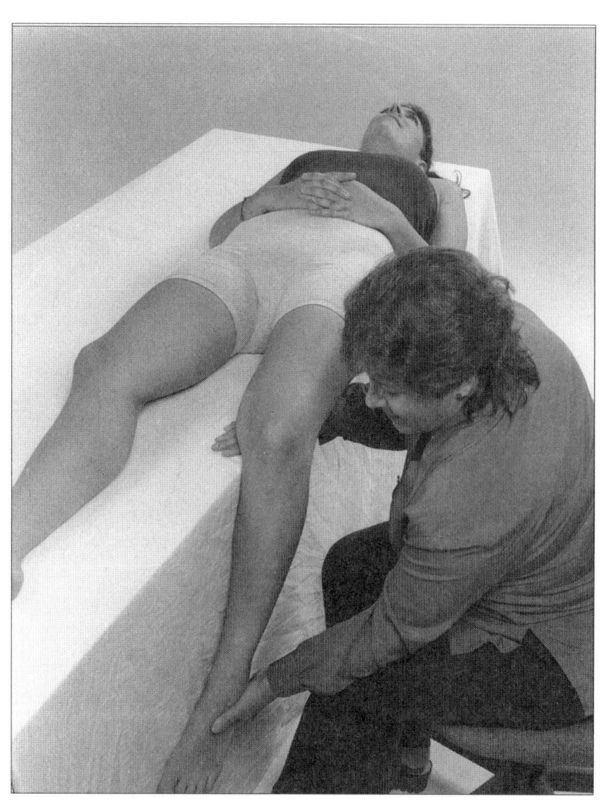

Medial Meniscus

Knee Dysfunction

EVALUATE

Point tenderness over joint line at medial aspect of joint. Evaluate flexion and extension.

TENDER POINT

On the medial meniscus.

TREATMENT

- Supine.
- Ipsilateral leg over the edge of the treatment table.
- Slight hip abduction (about 10 degrees) on the ipsilateral side.
- Knee flexion to 40 degrees on the ipsilateral side.
- Apply strong internal rotation force to the ipsilateral tibia with slight adduction of the tibia.

Posterior Cruciate

Knee Dysfunction

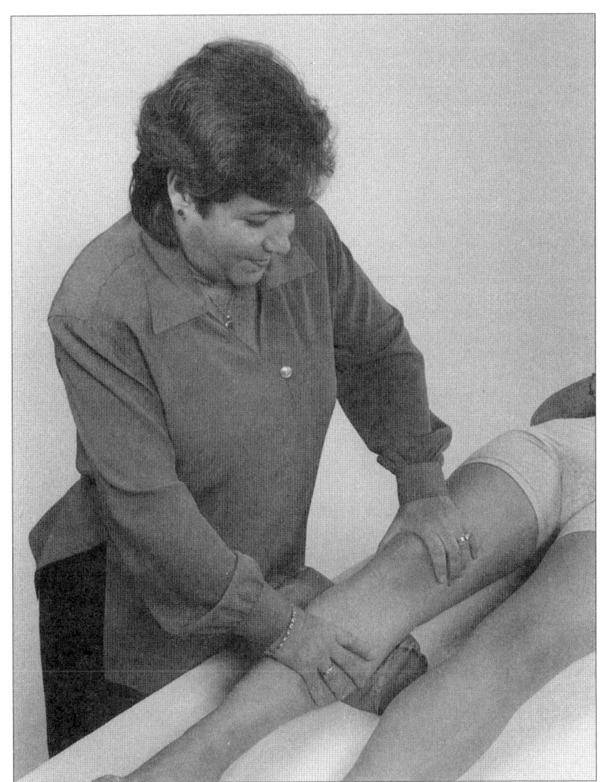

EVALUATE

Flexion and extension of the knee.

TENDER POINT

Middle of popliteal space.

TREATMENT

- Supine.
- Place a towel roll under the proximal end of the ipsilateral tibia.
- Apply an anterior to posterior force through the ipsilateral distal femur.
- Ipsilateral tibial internal rotation with overpressure.

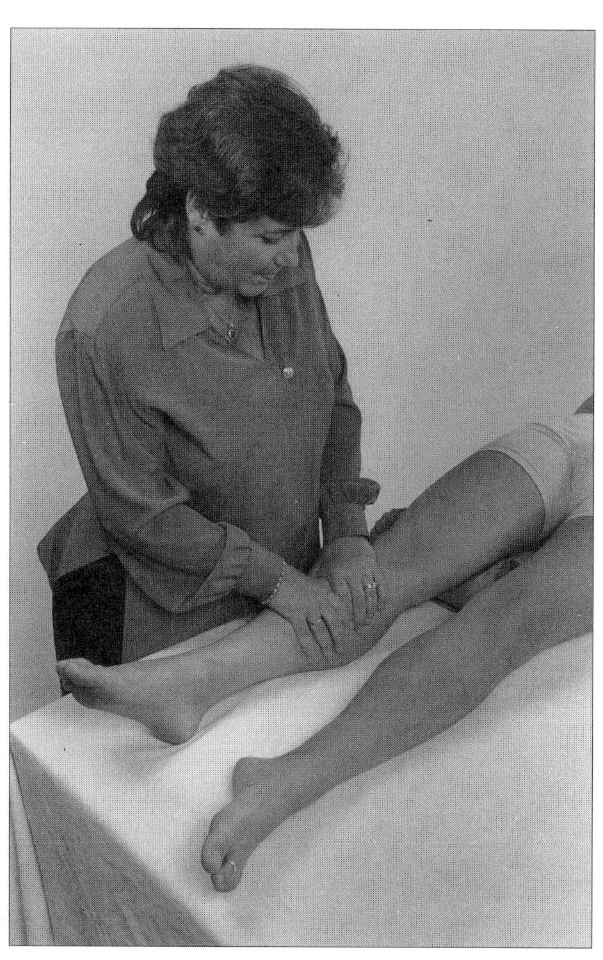

Anterior Cruciate

Knee Dysfunction

EVALUATE

Flexion and extension of the knee.

TENDER POINT

Hamstring muscle behind the knee in the popliteal region.

TREATMENT

- Supine.
- Place a towel roll under the ipsilateral distal end of the femur.
- Apply an anterior to posterior force through the ipsilateral proximal tibia.
- Therapist then applies an internal rotation with overpressure through the proximal tibia.

Medial Gastrocnemius

Foot/Ankle Dysfunction

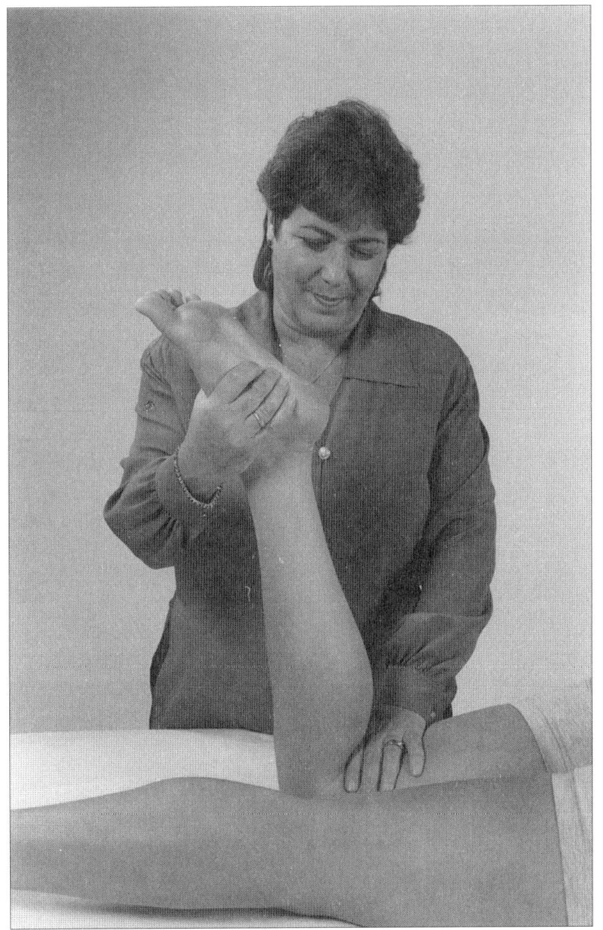

EVALUATE

Ankle dorsiflexion.

TENDER POINT

Medial third of posterior knee joint line, approximately half inch to 1 inch caudal.

TREATMENT

- Prone.
- Knee flexion to 90 degrees on the ipsilateral side.
- Internal rotation on the ipsilateral tibia with slight inversion on the foot.
- Add compression of the ipsilateral knee joint through the tibia.
- Plantar flexion with overpressure.
- **Synergic Pattern Release**

INTEGRATIVE MANUAL THERAPY

The influence of the gastrocnemius will often astonish the practitioner. The influence of the gastrocnemius is evident with the effects of Strain and Counterstrain Technique. The gastrocnemius performs plantar flexion; loss of dorsiflexion is extremely common, often caused by plantar flexor spasm. In the hemiplegic client, measurements of EMG studies have shown that prolonged and premature firing is a typical problem, affecting heel loading and weight bearing in stance phase. Compensation for loss of dorsiflexion which is secondary to gastrocnemius spasm is varied, and results may be profound. Calcaneal apophysitis, plantar fasciitis, shin splints, chondromalasia, and multiple other problems may subside in intensity and frequency after utilizing this technique.

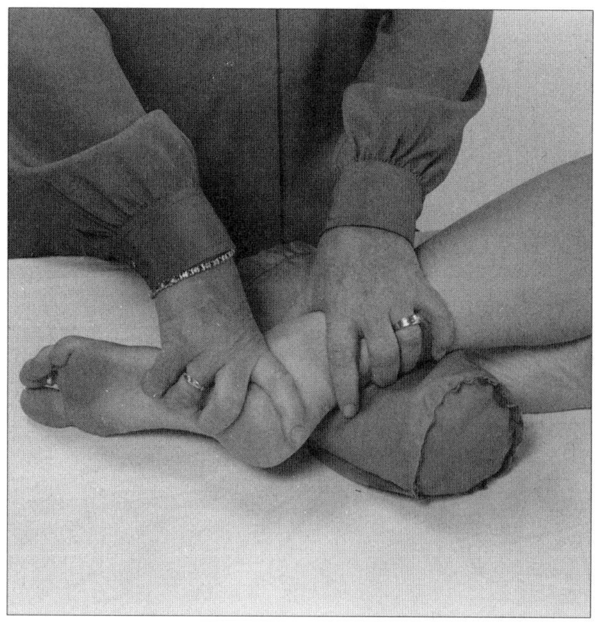

Medial Ankle

Foot/Ankle Dysfunction

EVALUATE

Eversion, abduction, pronation of the foot (non weight bearing), static foot posture.

TENDER POINT

2 cm below medial malleolus.

TREATMENT

- Side lying on contralateral side of Tender Point.
- Ipsilateral medial ankle (with Tender Point) facing floor.
- Foot and ankle are off table with a towel roll padding under the ankle.
- Knee flexion to 90 degrees on the ipsilateral side.
- Push from the lateral side of the talus downward towards the floor, causing a medial shear force of 2 to 5 pounds (medial shear of the talus).
- **Synergic Pattern Release**

INTEGRATIVE MANUAL THERAPY

The medial ankle technique (for the tibiotalar joint) and the medial calcaneal technique (for the subtalar joint) will reduce supination/varus deviations, i.e., the high arch foot. This technique is excellent to decrease frequency of ankle sprains.

Medial Calcaneus

Foot/Ankle Dysfunction

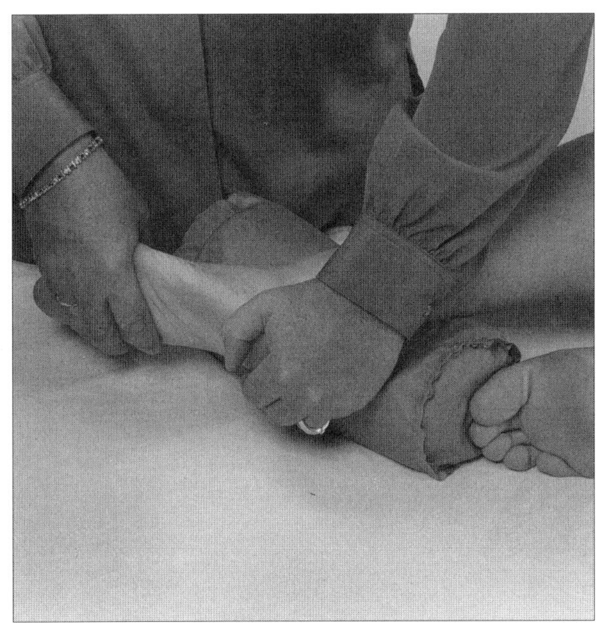

EVALUATE

Eversion, abduction, pronation of the foot (non-weight bearing), static foot posture.

TENDER POINT

3 cm caudal and posterior to medial malleolus.

TREATMENT

- Side lying on the contralateral side of Tender Point.
- Ipsilateral medial ankle facing floor.
- Apply up to 5 pounds force; push medial (towards the floor) on the calcaneus.
- Medial shear of calcaneus.
- Add a 1 pound counter-rotation force to the forefoot.
- **Synergic Pattern Release**

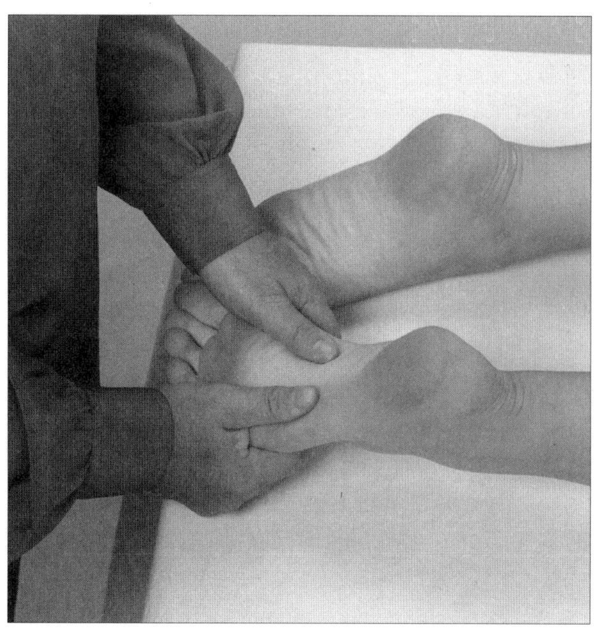

Talus

Foot/Ankle Dysfunction

EVALUATE

Dorsiflexion of the foot.

TENDER POINT

2 cm below medial malleolus and 2 cm anterior.

TREATMENT

- Prone.
- Turn the ipsilateral foot so that the medial aspect of the foot is facing up to the ceiling.
- Force the foot into marked inversion with overpressure with 1 pound internal rotation force on the foot.
- **Synergic Pattern Release**

INTEGRATIVE MANUAL THERAPY

The talus technique is excellent for treatment of the pronated, flat foot. The runner with shin splints will bless the practitioner who teaches him/her how to perform this technique at home with a friend or family member. Frequent cramps of the calf at night may subside. When an infant is born with club feet, the parents can be taught this technique, to perform daily, until the foot posture shows changes, after which time frequency may be decreased.

Flexed Calcaneus

Foot/Ankle Dysfunction

EVALUATE

Limitation of Motion: Passive mid foot flexibility and plantar fascia mobility.

TENDER POINT

Plantar surface of the foot at the anterior end of the calcaneus.

TREATMENT

- Prone.
- Knee flexion to 90 degrees on the ipsilateral side.
- Dorsum of the ipsilateral foot is pushed to attain hyper-plantar flexion.
- Apply force onto calcaneus. Push calcaneus towards the toes, into hyper-flexion.
- **Synergic Pattern Release**

INTEGRATIVE MANUAL THERAPY

This technique is excellent for plantar fasciitis. It can be used together with the medial ankle and medial calcaneal techniques.

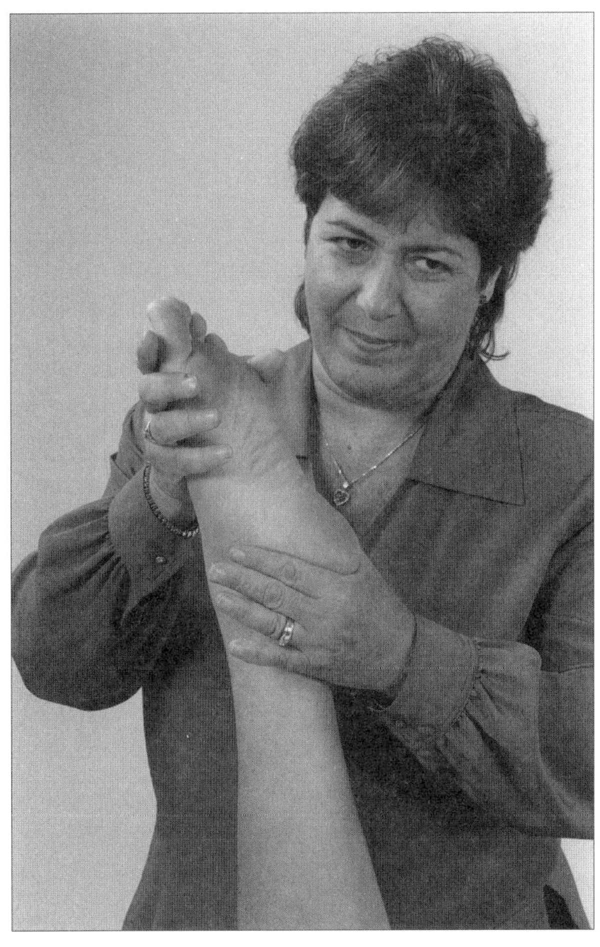

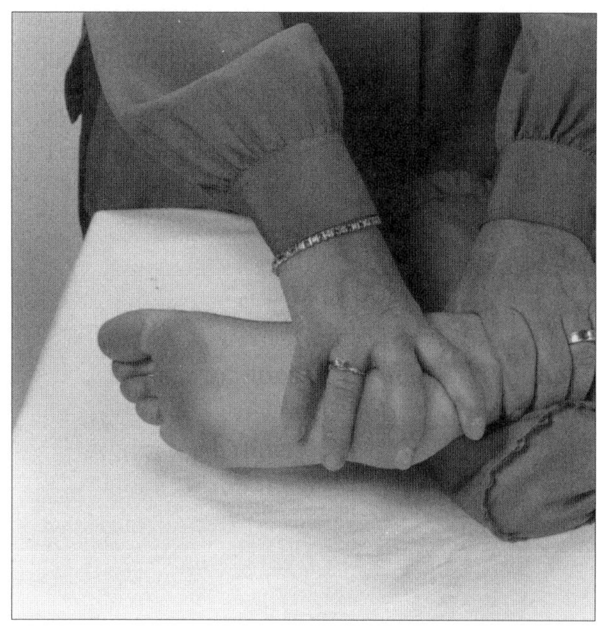

Lateral Ankle

Foot/Ankle Dysfunction

EVALUATE

Supination, inversion, adduction.

TENDER POINT

In front of lateral malleolus.

TREATMENT

- Sidelying on the ipsilateral side of the Tender Point.
- Tender Point towards the floor.
- Place a towel roll under the ipsilateral distal tibia.
- Apply a force onto talus. Talus is forced into lateral shear.
- Attain a lateral shear of talus.
- **Synergic Pattern Release**

INTEGRATIVE MANUAL THERAPY

This technique is excellent for tibio-fibular problems, problems of the anterior compartment of the shin and shin splints.

Lateral Calcaneus

Foot/Ankle Dysfunction

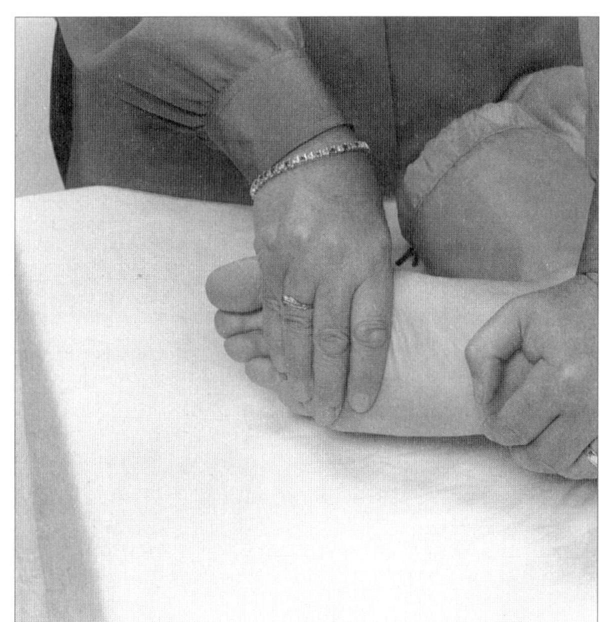

EVALUATE

Supination, inversion, adduction.

TENDER POINT

2 cm inferior and posterior to the lateral malleolus.

TREATMENT

- Sidelying on the ipsilateral side of the Tender Point.
- Tender Point towards the floor.
- Apply a lateral force onto the ipsilateral calcaneus. Shear the calcaneus lateral.
- The other hand counter-rotates the ipsilateral forefoot with 1 pound force.
- **Synergic Pattern Release**

CHAPTER 11

TREATMENT OF UPPER QUADRANT HYPERTONICITY

FOR SYNERGIC PATTERN RELEASE WITH STRAIN AND COUNTERSTRAIN TECHNIQUE

Brachial Plexus Compromise

The brachial plexus may be compressed. There are typical patho-anatomic sites of compression of the brachial plexus, contributing to the pain and paresthesia of the arm and hand. Spinal cord fibrosis of the cervical spinal cord and cervical nerve root impingement are contributing factors to brachial plexus compromise. Common sites of direct compression of the plexus include: between the middle and the anterior scalene muscles, which may be in spasm secondary to cervical or other problems; within the costoclavicular joint space, between clavicle and the first rib; underneath the pectoralis minor, which may be in spasm because of rib cage and intrathoracic problems; and in axilla, compressed by a caudal humeral head.

The intention of the following tests is to isolate the patho-anatomic sites of compression of the client, and to adapt therapy so that the compromise of the plexus is alleviated. The Strain and Counterstrain points which are exceptionally valuable are listed with the test.

If there is compression between the scalene muscles, treat with the lateral and anterior cervical Strain and Counterstrain techniques. Then apply a lateral neck hold, and perform the Soft Tissue Myofascial Release technique to further decrease signs and symptoms.

If the test for compromise of the plexus under the pectoralis minor is positive, treat with the second depressed rib technique. Then perform a Soft Tissue Myofascial Release technique to the clavipectoral fascia.

Another site of compression may be within axilla, compromised by pressure from an inferior displacement of the humeral head. The Strain and Counterstrain technique for the latissimus dorsi can be performed. The latissimus dorsi is the depressor of the humeral head, and may cause compression of the brachial plexus in axilla.

The following assessments (1, 2, 3) will determine where treatment would be most effective:

Assessment 1

Test to Compromise the Middle and Anterior Scalene Compression of the Brachial Plexus

1. Flex the occipito-atlantal joint (chin tuck).
2. Rotate the head towards the compromised side maintaining occipito-atlantal flexion.

TREATMENT

Strain and Counterstrain: Lateral Cervicals for the Middle Scalenes; Anterior Cervicals (4 through 7) for the Anterior Scalenes.

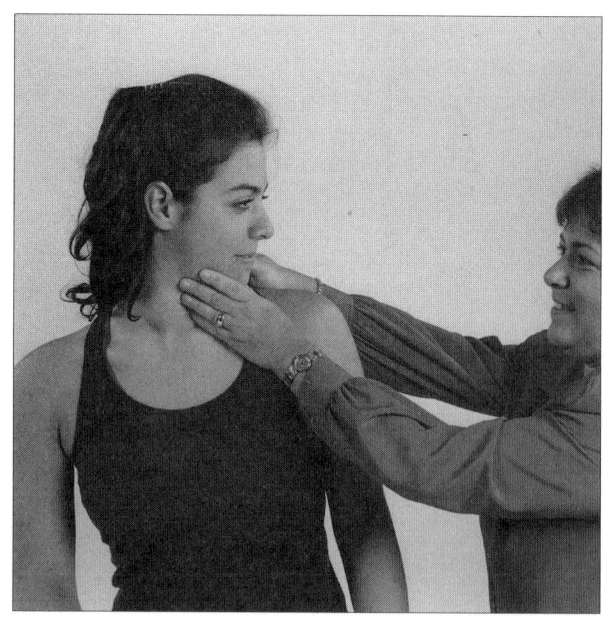

Assessment 2

Test to Compromise the Costoclavicular Joint Compression of the Brachial Plexus

1. Place longitudinal traction on the arm.
2. Inhale and maintain inspiration.
3. Resist elevation of the shoulder girdle (shoulder shrugging).

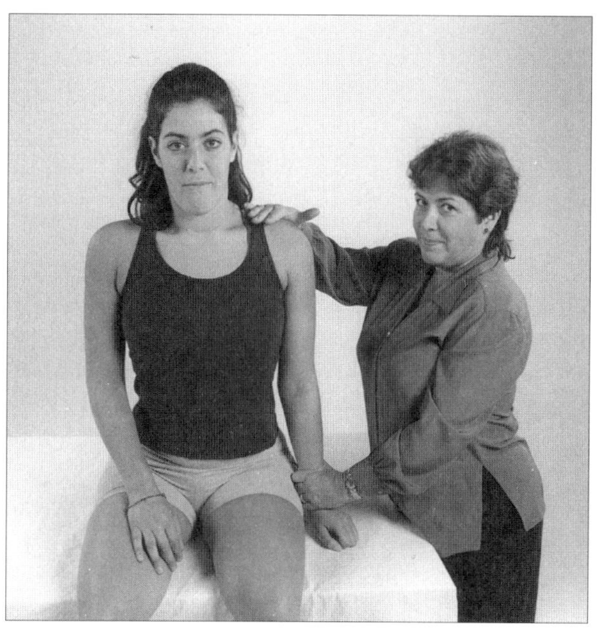

TREATMENT

Strain and Counterstrain: Anterior First Thoracic; Anterior Seventh/Eighth Cervical; Anterior Acromioclavicular; Posterior Acromioclavicular; Elevated First Rib; Lateral Cervicals.

Assessment 3

Test to Compromise the Pectoralis Minor Compression of the Brachial Plexus

1. Extend the arm with external rotation.
2. Maintain passive shoulder extension with external rotation.
3. Resist shoulder girdle protraction.

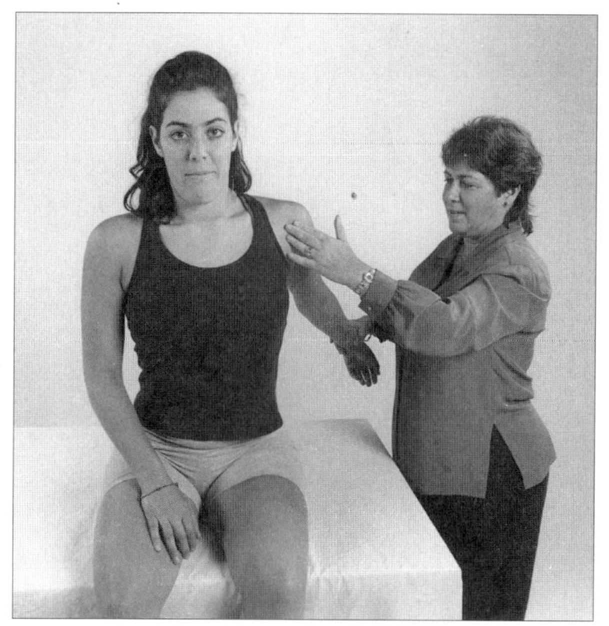

TREATMENT

- Strain and Counterstrain: Second Depressed Rib (pectoralis minor).

INTEGRATIVE MANUAL THERAPY

If there is compression between the scalene muscles, apply a lateral neck hold, and perform the Soft Tissue Myofascial Release Technique to further decrease signs and symptoms. If the test for compromise of the plexus under the pectoralis minor is positive, treat with a Soft Tissue Myofascial Release Technique to the clavipectoral fascia. Another site of compression may be within axilla compromised by pressure from an inferior displacement of the humeral head. The Strain and Counterstrain for the latissimus dorsi can be performed. The latissimus dorsi is the depressor of the humeral head, and may cause compression of the brachial plexus in axilla.

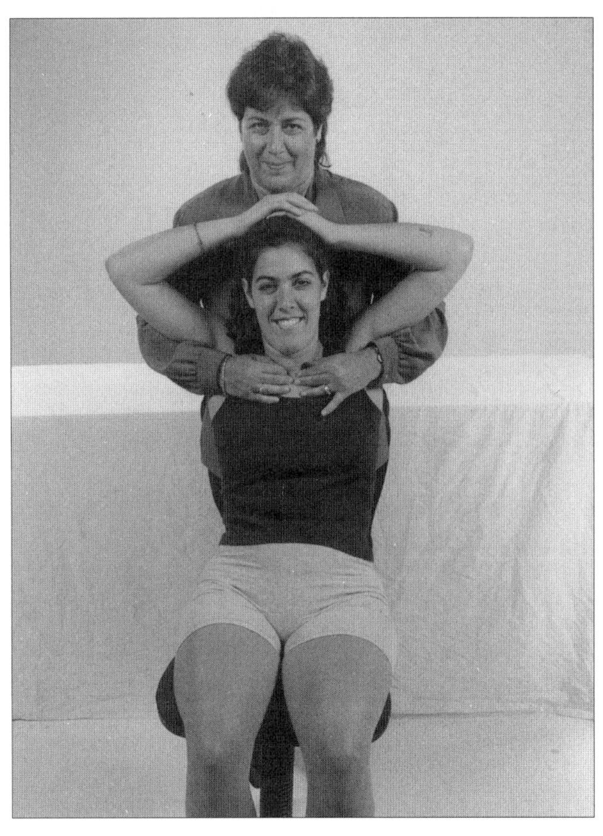

Anterior First Thoracic (AT1)

Thoracic Spine Dysfunction

EVALUATE

Limitation of Motion: Thoracic extension (hyperkyphosis), segmental movement.

TENDER POINT

Midline at the suprasternal notch.

TREATMENT

- Sitting.
- Do not lean on the patient's neck.
- Patient's hands behind head.
- Flex the client to T1.
- Slide buttocks forward on chair, keeping neck perpendicular to the floor, i.e., flexing up the spine.
- **Synergic Pattern Release**

INTEGRATIVE MANUAL THERAPY

This is the most valuable Strain and Counterstrain technique for the thoracic inlet. The anterior shear of T1 will cause the "dowager's hump." Drainage problems of lymph and venous systems will occur secondary to the dysfunction caused by this spasm.

Third and Fourth Anterior Thoracic (AT3, AT4)

Thoracic Spine Dysfunction

EVALUATE

Limitation of Motion: Thoracic extension (hyperkyphosis), segmental movement.

TENDER POINT

AT3: On sternum, 1 inch inferior to sterno-manubrial joint line.
AT4: On sternum, 2 inches inferior to sterno-manubrial joint line.

TREATMENT

- Sitting.
- Patient's two arms extended.
- Flex the client to T4.
- Slide buttocks forward on chair, keeping neck perpendicular to the floor, i.e., flexing up the spine.

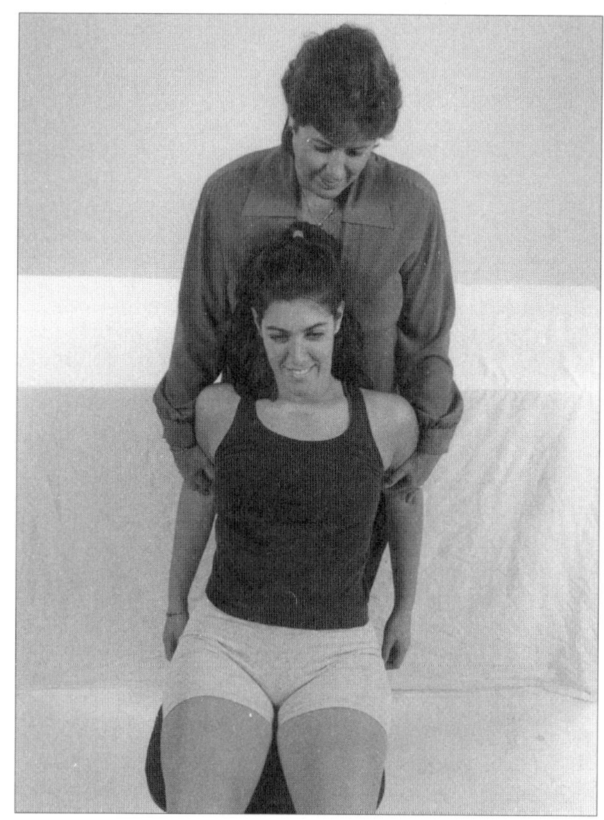

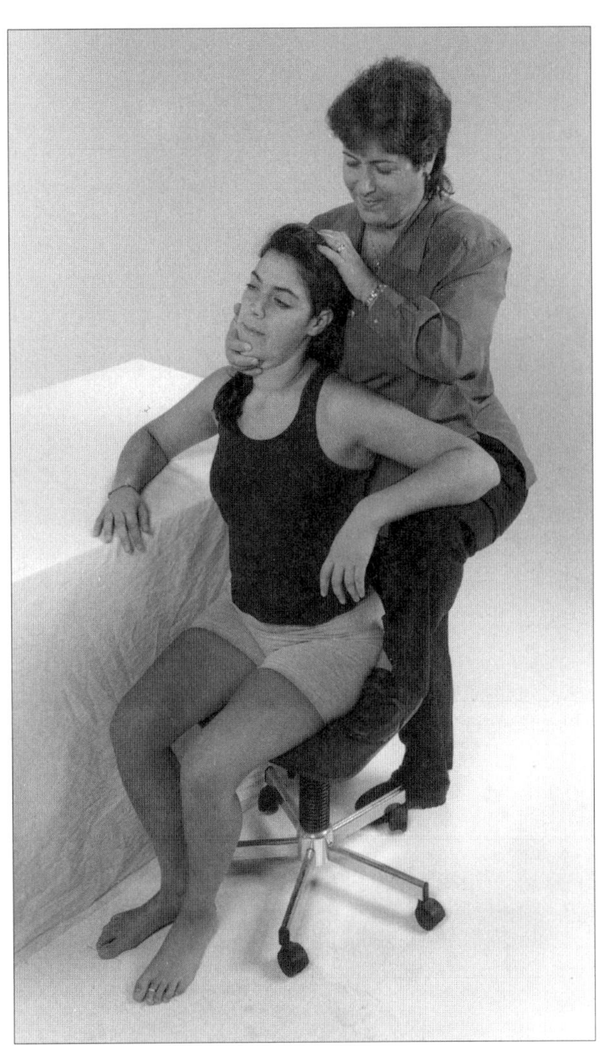

First Elevated Rib

Rib Cage Dysfunction

EVALUATE

Limitation of Motion: Cervicothoracic side bending and rotation, upper costal breathing.

TENDER POINT

Beneath margin of Trapezius at side of neck.

TREATMENT

- Sitting.
- Support ipsilateral shoulder (as shown in photograph)
- Slight head extension (less than 10 degrees) with "chin tuck."
- Slight cervical side bend (less than 10 degrees) on the ipsilateral side.
- Cervical rotation to the contralateral side.
- **Synergic Pattern Release**

Depressed Second Rib (Pectoralis Minor)

Rib Cage Dysfunction

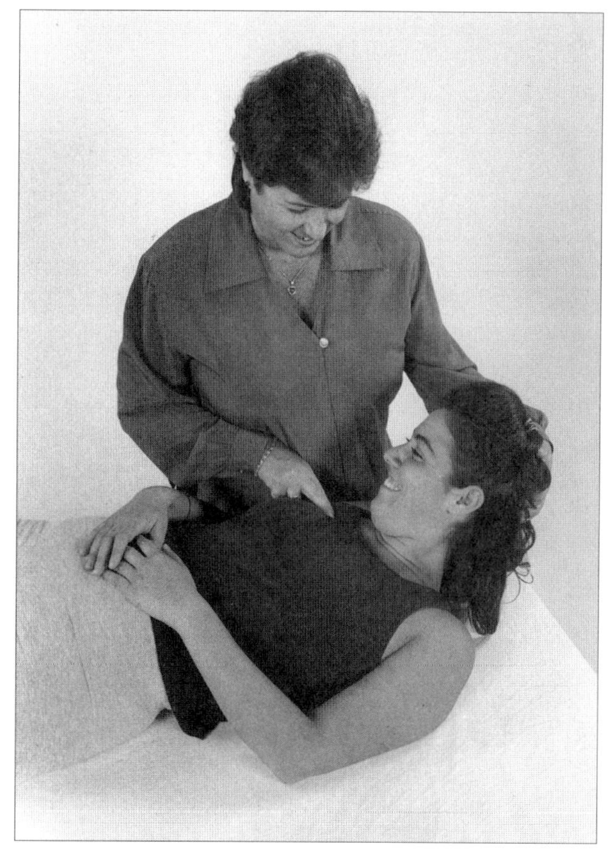

EVALUATE

Limitation of Motion: Shoulder girdle retraction and horizontal abduction, upper costal breathing.

TENDER POINT

Midway on a line between sternoclavicular joint and axilla.

TREATMENT

- Supine.
- Flex head and neck to end of range without overpressure.
- Point nose directly towards Tender Point. This will attain rotation and sidebending as required.
- **Synergic Pattern Release**

INTEGRATIVE MANUAL THERAPY

The second depressed rib is because of spasm of the pectoralis minor muscle, which originates from the second, third and fourth ribs, and inserts on the coracoid process. The most significant postural deviation caused by the pectoralis minor is the protracted shoulder girdle.

---

*Integration: This technique will address the shoulder girdle protraction component of the typical synergic pattern.

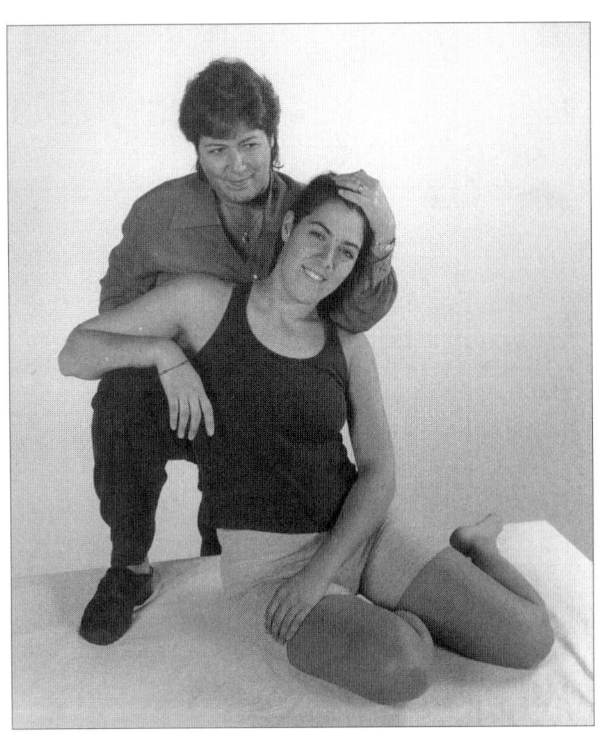

Elevated Ribs

Rib Cage Dysfunction

EVALUATE

Limitation of Motion: Thoracic side bending to ipsilateral side (segmental movement), rib excursion.

TENDER POINT

Posterior on angle of rib.

TREATMENT

- Side sitting.
- Place the client's feet on the contralateral side of the treated ribs.
- Further elevate an already elevated rib.
- Side bend to the contralateral side, to the rib being treated.

Depressed Ribs

Rib Cage Dysfunction

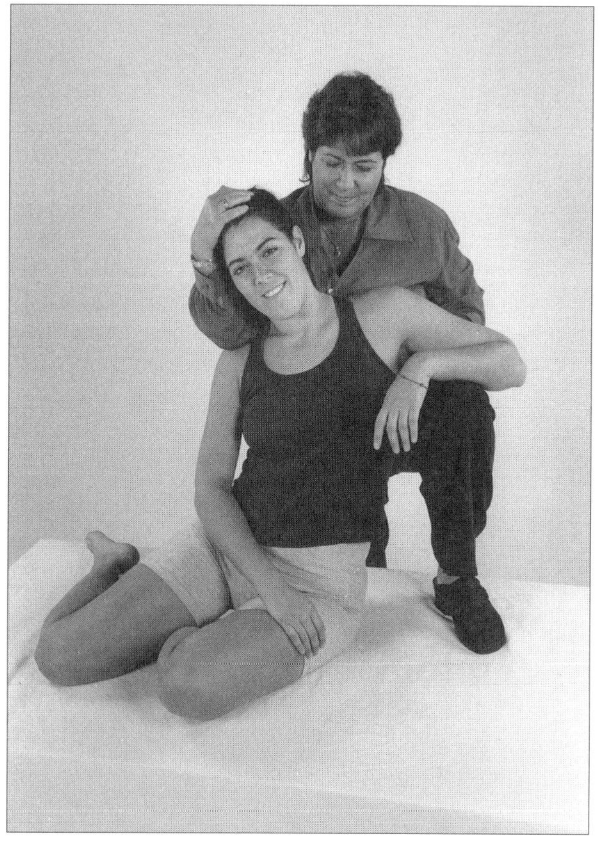

EVALUATE

Limitation of Motion: Thoracic side bending to opposite side (segmental movement).

TENDER POINT

On ribs, midaxillary line and slightly anterior for lower ribs.

TREATMENT

- Side sitting.
- Place the client's feet on the ipsilateral side of the treated rib.
- Further depress the already depressed rib.
- Side bend towards the ipsilateral side, to the rib being treated.

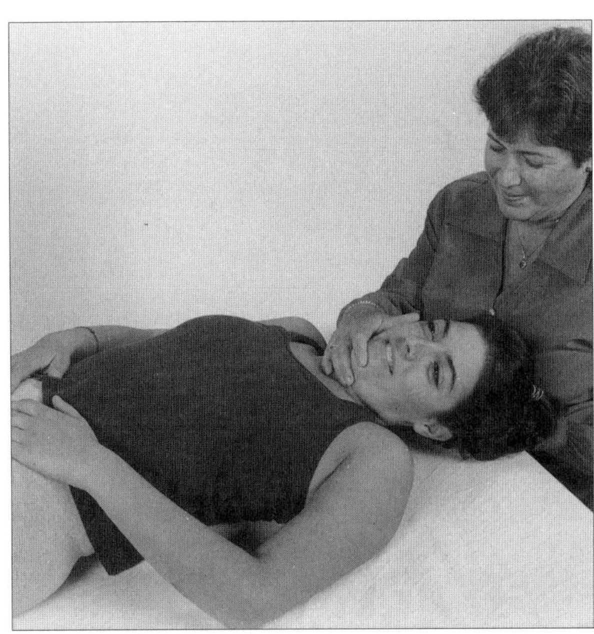

Anterior First Cervical

Dysfunction of the Neck

EVALUATE

Limitation of Motion: Cervical extension, segmental movement. (Beware of anterior cervical shears: maintain segmental movement.)

TENDER POINT

Posterior surface of ascending ramus of mandible under ear.

TREATMENT

- Supine.
- Support occiput.
- Slight cervical flexion. (Chin tuck.)
- Significant cervical rotation to 60 degrees on the contralateral side of the Tender Point.
- Slight cervical side bend to 10 degrees on the contralateral side of the Tender Point.

Anterior Third Cervical

Dysfunction of the Neck

EVALUATE

Limitation of Motion: Cervical Extension, segmental movement. (Beware of anterior cervical shears: maintain segmental movement.)

TENDER POINT

Anterior tip of transverse process of C3.

TREATMENT

- Supine.
- Minimal cervical flexion to 20 degrees.
- Apply traction.
- Relax and enhance chin tuck.
- Ipsilateral cervical side bend to 15 degrees.

INTEGRATIVE MANUAL THERAPY

The anterior cervical Strain and Counterstrain techniques are all valuable, and can be performed as a group: anterior third cervical, anterior fourth cervical, anterior fifth cervical. The flexors of the cervical spine are always in a state of hypertonicity, The hyoid muscles are maintained on stretch because of the cervical flexion. Swallowing and articulation problems are common. These techniques can help improve speech and oral-motor function.

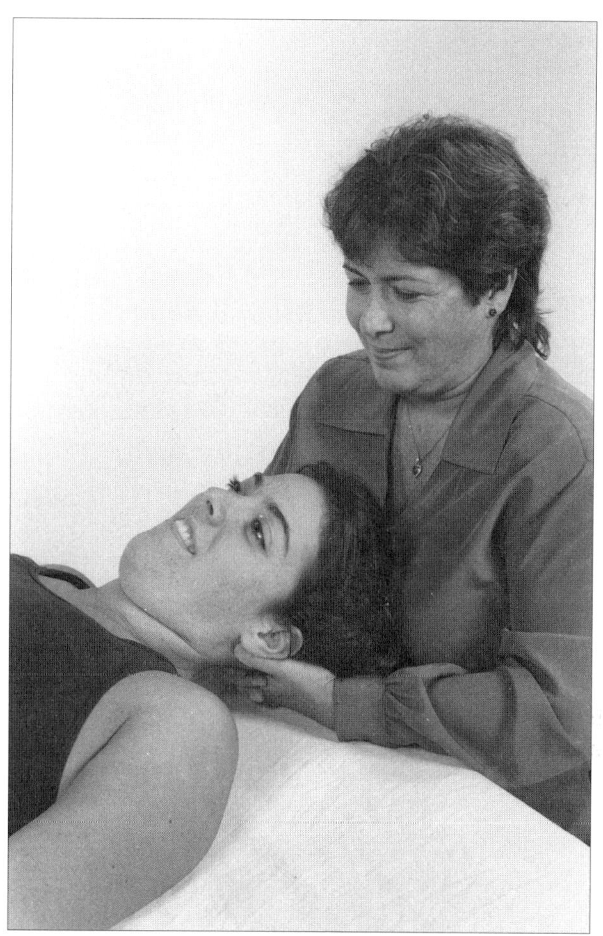

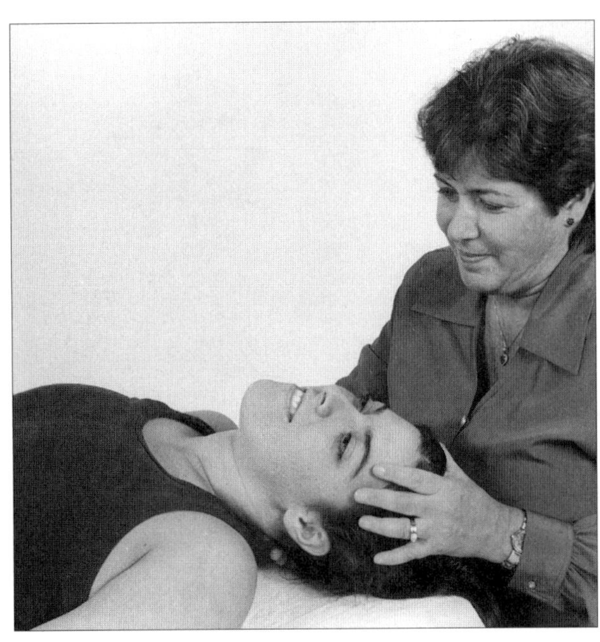

Anterior Fourth Cervical

Dysfunction of the Neck

EVALUATE

Limitation of Motion: Cervical extension, segmental movement. (Beware of anterior cervical shears: maintain segmental movement.)

TENDER POINT

Anterior tip of transverse process of C4.

TREATMENT

- Supine.
- Slight extension. (Place index finger under C4. Push/displace C4 in anterior direction.)
- Contralateral cervical rotation to 20 degrees to the Tender Point.
- Contralateral cervical side bending to 20 degrees to the Tender Point.

Anterior Fifth Cervical

Dysfunction of the Neck

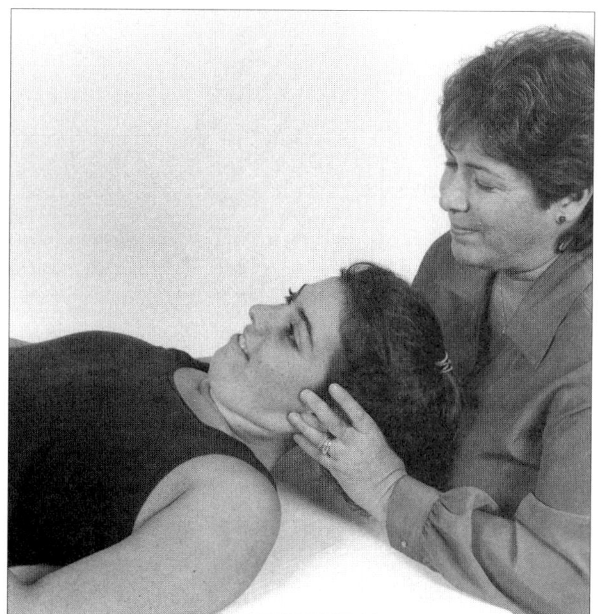

EVALUATE

Limitation of Motion: Cervical extension, segmental movement. (Beware of anterior cervical shears: maintain segmental movement.)

TENDER POINT

Anterior surface of tip of transverse process of C5.

TREATMENT

- Supine.
- Cervical flexion to C5 (about 45 degrees).
- Contralateral cervical rotation to 25 degrees to the Tender Point.
- Contralateral cervical side bending to 25 degrees to the Tender Point.

INTEGRATIVE MANUAL THERAPY

This technique is as valuable for first aid as the Anterior Fifth Lumbar Technique. When the right anterior of C5 is in spasm, C5 is stuck flexed, rotated right and side bent right. As a result of this static position, the hydrostatic pressure on the C5 disc will be influenced, and the C5 disc will protrude, posterior and to the left. The intradiscal pressure will increase because of the rotation of C5. Compromise of the left C5 nerve root can occur secondary to the pressure of the protruding disc. Compromise of the right C5 nerve root can be secondary to the closure of the right facet joint because of the position of the C5 vertebra. Cervical syndrome is markedly improved with this technique.

---

*Integration: This technique will address cervical discopathy and referred shoulder pain.

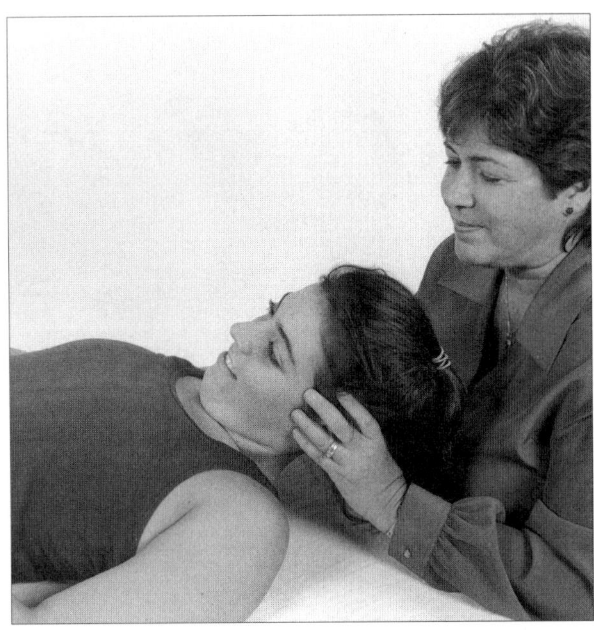

Anterior Seventh Cervical

Dysfunction of the Neck

EVALUATE

Limitation of Motion: Cervical extension, segmental movement. (Beware of anterior cervical shears: maintain segmental movement.)

TENDER POINT

Posterosuperior surface of clavicle, 3 cm lateral to medial end.

TREATMENT

- Supine.
- Cervical flexion to C7 (about 55 degrees).
- Contralateral cervical rotation to 40 degrees to the Tender Point.
- Contralateral cervical side bend to 40 degrees to the Tender Point.
- **Synergic Pattern Release**

INTEGRATIVE MANUAL THERAPY

The anterior seventh and eighth cervical Strain and Counterstrain techniques are for the sternocleidomastoid muscles. Torticollis may be improved with these techniques. Because the SCM inserts on the temporal bones, often tinnitus and other ear symptoms can occur secondary to this dysfunction.

Anterior Eighth Cervical

Dysfunction of the Neck

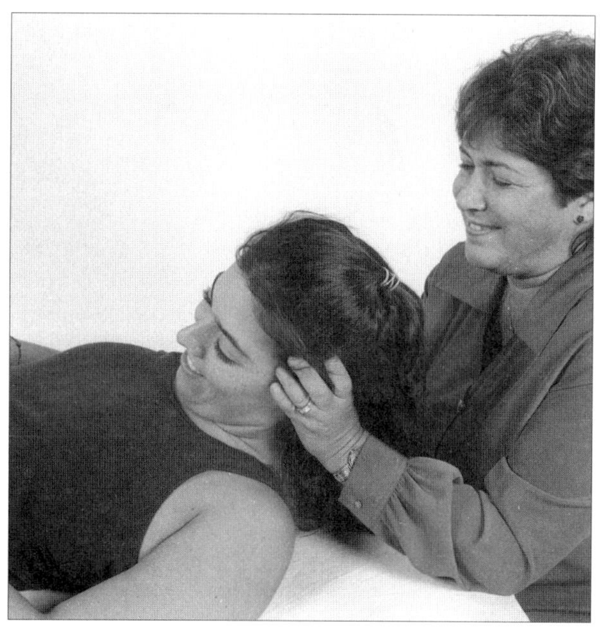

EVALUATE

Limitation of Motion: Cervical extension, segmental movement. (Beware of anterior cervical shears: maintain segmental movement.)

TENDER POINT

Medial end of clavicle.

TREATMENT

- Supine.
- Cervical flexion to C8 interspace (about 50 to 60 degrees).
- Apply traction.
- Contralateral cervical rotation to 60 degrees to the Tender Point.
- Contralateral cervical side bending to 60 degrees to the Tender Point.

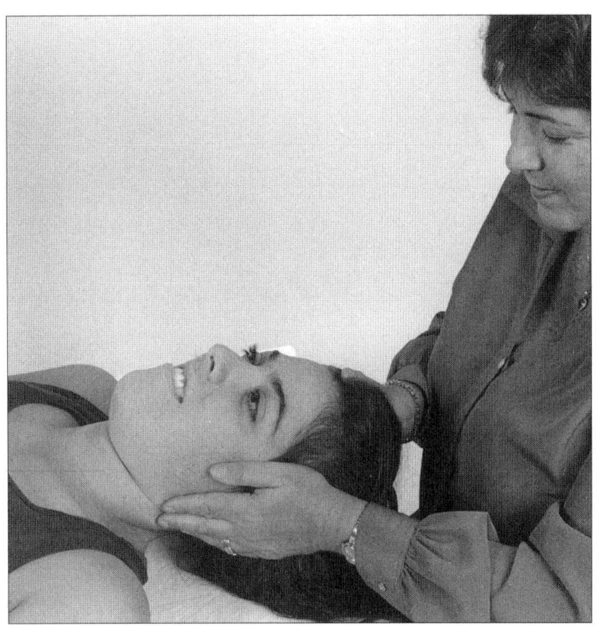

Lateral Cervicals

Dysfunction of the Neck

EVALUATE

Limitation of Motion: Cervical side bending to opposite side, segmental movement. Lateral cervical shears.

TENDER POINT

On the lateral tip of the transverse process.

TREATMENT

- Supine.
- Cervical side bending to the specific cervical segment ipsilateral to the Tender Point.
- Cervical rotation to the specific cervical segment ipsilateral to the Tender Point.
- Therapist places the contralateral hand, to the client's Tender Point, on the client's contralateral parietal bone.
- Therapist places the ipsilateral hand, to the client's Tender Point, on the client's ipsilateral lower lateral face/mandible.
- Add *overpressure* to attain side glide at that segment.
- Place the opposite hand on the opposite parietal.
- The hand on the side of the Tender Point is on the lower lateral face/mandible.
- Compress the therapist's hands bilaterally to attain an ipsilateral side glide/hyper side bending effect.
- **Synergic Pattern Release**

INTEGRATIVE MANUAL THERAPY

The lateral cervical Strain and Counterstrain techniques will decrease the spasm of the middle scalene muscles. Often brachial plexus compromise is secondary to scalene spasm. The side bending and rotation of the vertebra which results from scalene spasm can contribute to discogenic problems. The vertebral artery will often become compromised within the foramina secondary to the tension of the scalene muscles.

---

*Integration: Thoracic Outlet Syndrome: To decrease brachial plexus compression between middle and anterior scalenes.

Posterior Cervicals

Dysfunction of the Neck

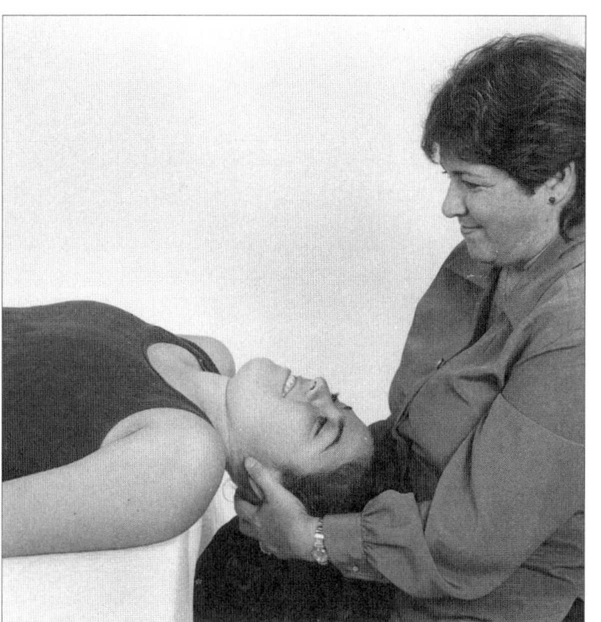

EVALUATE

Limitation of Motion: Cervical flexion, segmental movement.

TENDER POINT

On the spinous process or facet.

TREATMENT

- Supine.
- Head and neck to mid-scapula off the edge of the table.
- Extend the neck down the kinetic chain to the cervical segment.
- Ipsilateral cervical side bend and rotation down the kinetic chain towards the Tender Point.

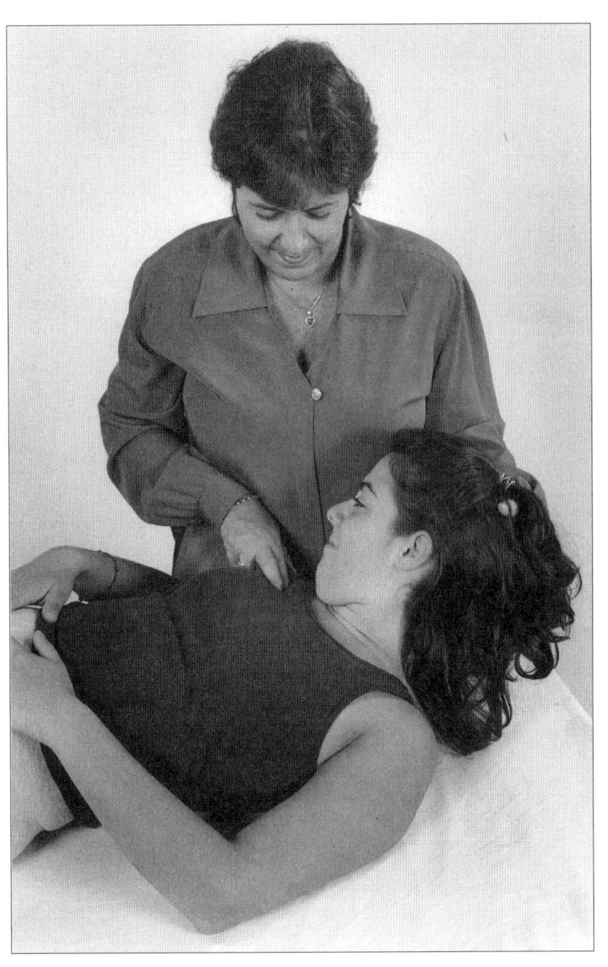

Depressed Second Rib (Pectoralis Minor)

The Protracted Shoulder Girdle

EVALUATE

Limitation of Motion: Horizontal abduction.

TENDER POINT

On the pectoralis minor, midpoint on an imaginary line between the sternoclavicular joint and axilla.

TREATMENT

- Supine.
- Flex head and neck to end of range without overpressure.
- Point nose directly towards Tender Point to attain rotation and side bending.
- **Synergic Pattern Release**

Anterior Acromioclavicular Joint

The Protracted Shoulder Girdle

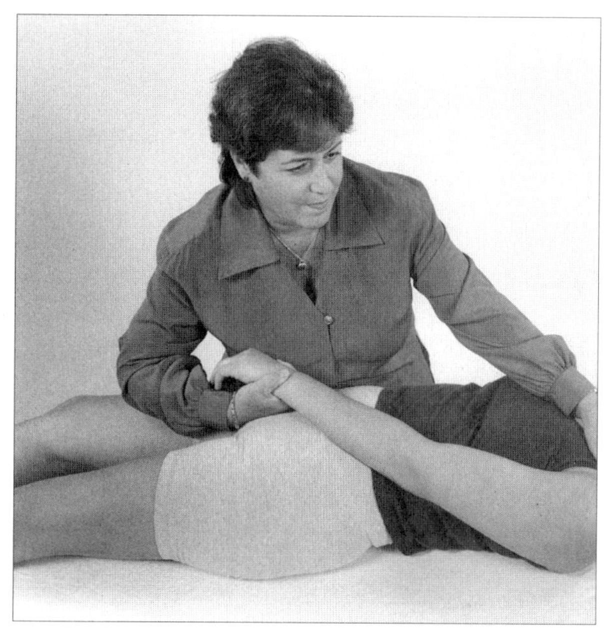

EVALUATE

Limitation of Motion: Shoulder joint external and internal rotation.

TENDER POINT

Anterior aspect of the distal clavicle.

TREATMENT

- Supine.
- Bring the client's ipsilateral hand, to the Tender Point, directly to the contralateral knee. Ipsilateral arm rests on anterior aspect of the body.
- Forcefully distract arm longitudinally, with 2 to 5 pounds force.
- **Synergic Pattern Release**

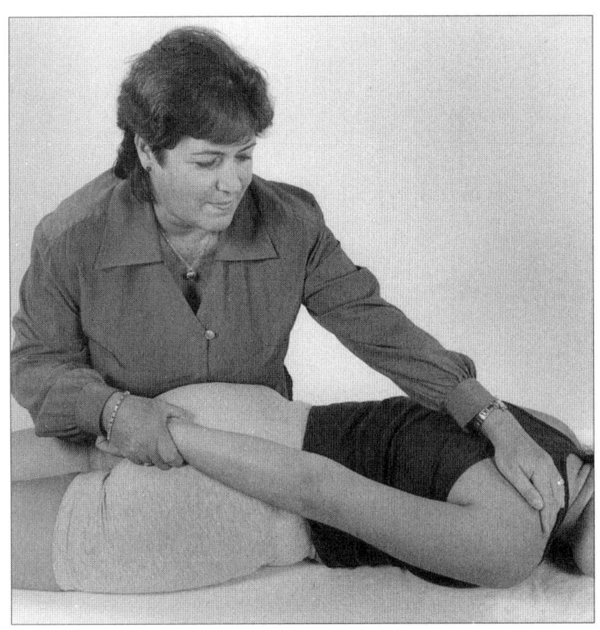

Posterior Acromioclavicular Joint

The Protracted Shoulder Girdle

EVALUATE

Limitation of Motion: Shoulder joint external and internal shoulder.

TENDER POINT

Posterolateral aspect of superior acromion.

TREATMENT

- Prone.
- Bring the client's ipsilateral hand, to the Tender Point, directly to the contralateral knee. Ipsilateral arm rests on posterior aspect of the body.
- Forcefully distract arm longitudinally, with 2 to 5 pounds force.
- **Synergic Pattern Release**

Third Depressed Rib and Frozen Shoulder

Upper Extremity Dysfunction

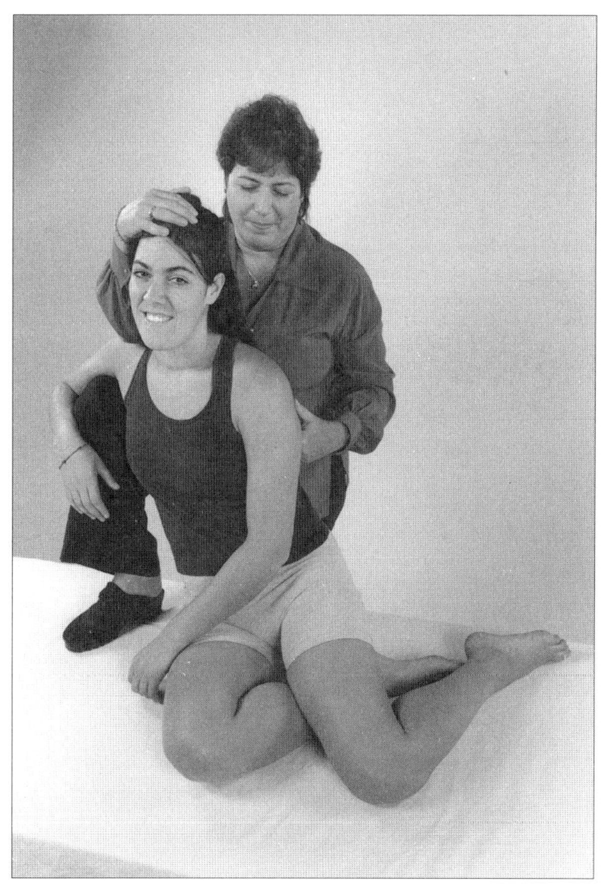

EVALUATE

Limitation of Motion: Shoulder Abduction.

TENDER POINT

On rib deep in axilla on midaxillary line.

TREATMENT

- Side sitting with client's feet to the ipsilateral side of the Tender Point.
- Ipsilateral side bending of the cervical and upper thoracic spine.

INTEGRATIVE MANUAL THERAPY

Neurointegration: These techniques will attain a decrease in the hypertonicity which contributes to the typical synergic pattern of spasticity, increased joint mobility and increased ranges of motion.

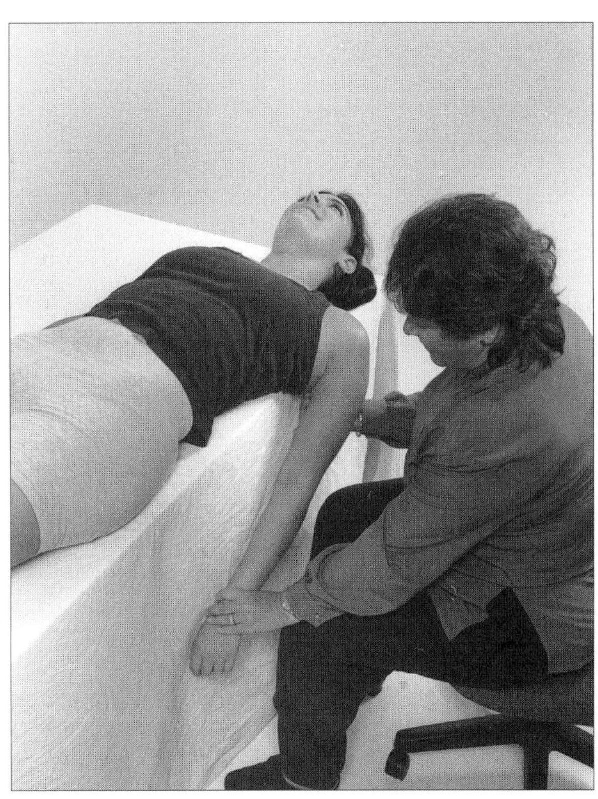

Subscapularis

Upper Extremity Dysfunction

EVALUATE

Limitation of Motion: Shoulder external rotation and abduction.

TENDER POINT

Deep into axilla on anterior aspect of humerus.

TREATMENT

- Supine.
- Ipsilateral arm off the bed.
- Ipsilateral shoulder extension to the end of range without overpressure.
- Ipsilateral shoulder internal rotation.
- Ipsilateral shoulder adduction with overpressure.
- **Synergic Pattern Release**

INTEGRATIVE MANUAL THERAPY

The subscapularis will cause the internal rotation of the glenohumeral joint whenever there is muscle spasm. Its most problematic contribution is the anterior shear/ subluxation of the humeral head. This problem at the shoulder joint is secondary in significance only to the inferior subluxation caused by the latissimus dorsi spasm. The sequence of treatment is as follows: (1) Second depressed rib (pectoralis minor); (2) Subscapularis; (3) Latissimus dorsi.

Infraspinatus (TS3)

Upper Extremity Dysfunction

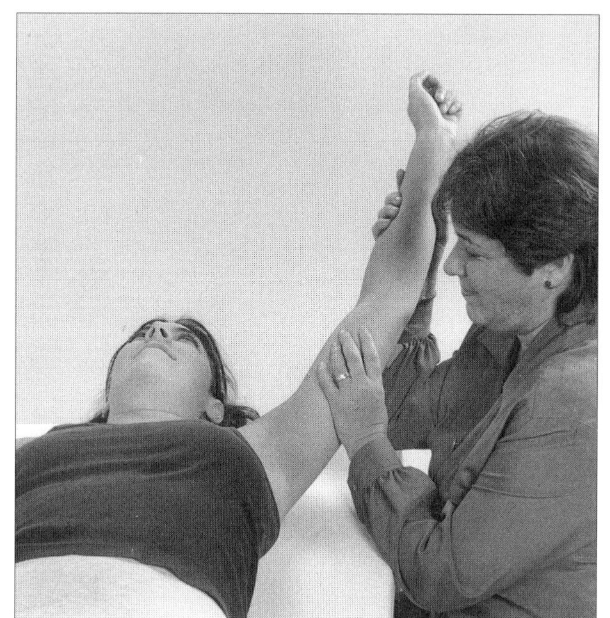

EVALUATE

Limitation of Motion: Shoulder internal rotation and scapulothoracic mobility.

TENDER POINT

5 cm beneath spine of scapula and 2 cm lateral to medial border.

TREATMENT

- Supine.
- Ipsilateral shoulder flexion to 135 degrees (with almost straight arm).

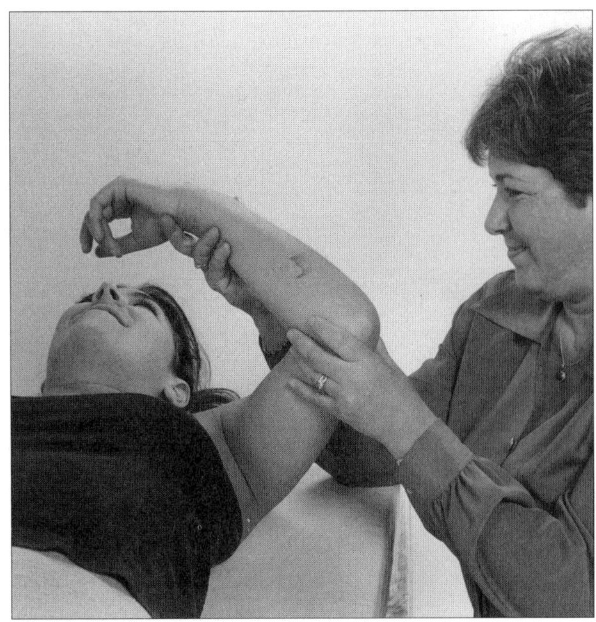

Supraspinatus (SP1)

Upper Extremity Dysfunction

EVALUATE

Limitation of Motion: Shoulder girdle depression and glenohumeral joint mobility.

TENDER POINT

Supraspinatus fossa 1 inch medial to acromioclavicular joint.

TREATMENT

- Supine.
- Ipsilateral shoulder flexion to 45 degrees.
- Ipsilateral shoulder abduction to 45 degrees.
- Ipsilateral shoulder external rotation to 45 degrees.
- **Synergic Pattern Release**

INTEGRATIVE MANUAL THERAPY

The diagnosis of supraspinatus tendinitis is common. This occurs secondary to friction of the tendon under the acromion, secondary to an abnormal vector of pull because of muscle spasm. The supraspinatus is also the major compressor of the humeral head, and causes significant osteoarthritic problems over a long period of hypertonicity.

Latissimus Dorsi

Upper Extremity Dysfunction

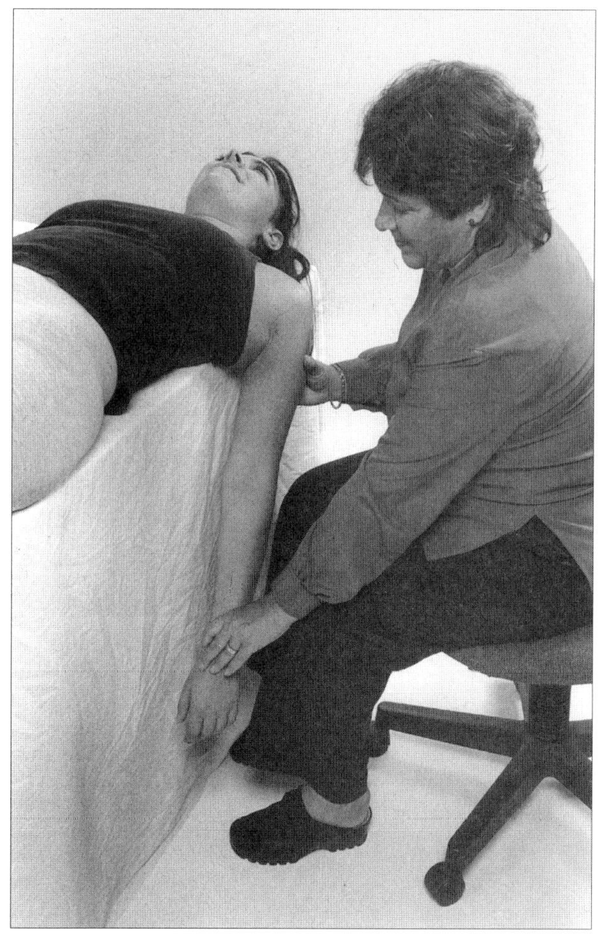

EVALUATE

Limitation of Motion: Shoulder flexion and elevation.

TENDER POINT

Deep into axilla on medial (posterior) aspect of humerus.

TREATMENT

- Supine.
- Ipsilateral arm off the bed.
- Ipsilateral shoulder extension to the end of range without overpressure.
- Ipsilateral shoulder adduction to end of range.
- Ipsilateral shoulder internal rotation to end of range.
- Ipsilateral arm is pulled with 5 pounds of longitudinal traction force.
- **Synergic Pattern Release**

INTEGRATIVE MANUAL THERAPY

This is the most valuable Strain and Counterstrain technique for the shoulder girdle. The latissimus dorsi is the only depressor of the humeral head, and is the major cause of inferior subluxation of the glenohumeral joint. Easy to correct with this technique, but the sequence is important. First perform the second depressed rib technique to eliminate the pectoralis minor spasm and reduce the protraction of the shoulder girdle. Next perform the subscapularis technique, so that the arm will be able to attain the extension required for the latissimus dorsi technique.

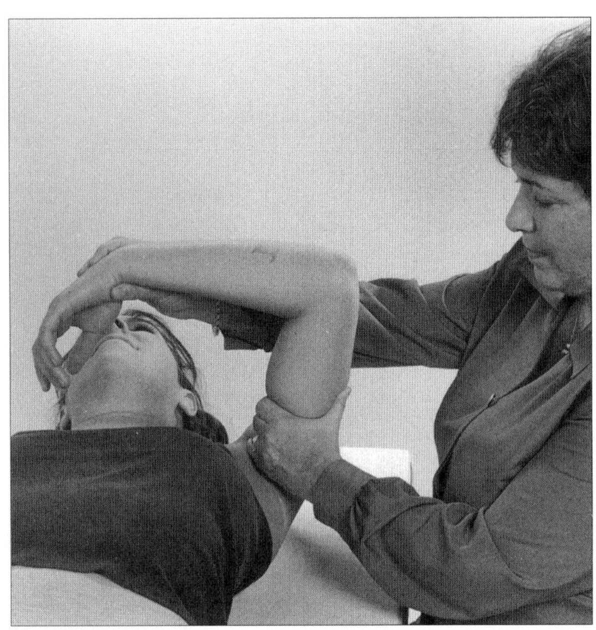

Biceps (Long Head)

Upper Extremity Dysfunction

EVALUATE

Limitation of Motion: Elbow extension.

TENDER POINT

Anterior surface of glenohumeral joint 1 inch superior to axilla.

TREATMENT

- Supine.
- Ipsilateral shoulder flexion to 90 degrees.
- Support forearm with 90 degrees flexion at elbow towards internal rotation.
- **Synergic Pattern Release**

INTEGRATIVE MANUAL THERAPY

When the biceps are in spasm there is often elbow pain, shoulder pain and wrist pain. Bicipital tendinitis will disappear with this technique, but it is necessary to treat proximal to distal, and first alleviate the muscle spasm of the more proximal musculature.

Radial Head (RAD)

Upper Extremity Dysfunction

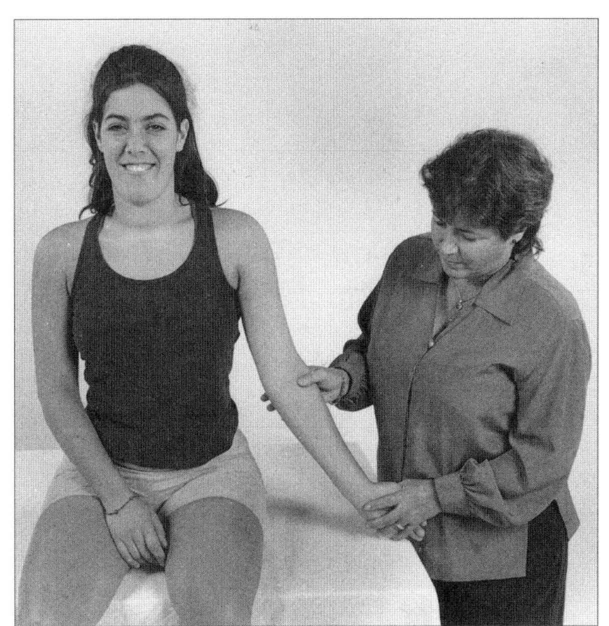

EVALUATE

Limitation of Motion: Elbow joint.

TENDER POINT

Anterolateral surface of head of radius.

TREATMENT

- Sitting or supine.
- Treatment in full ipsilateral elbow extension (no force).
- Supination and Abduction (slight force).
- **Synergic Pattern Release**

INTEGRATIVE MANUAL THERAPY

This is the major technique for tennis elbow, especially for the common etiology of brachioradialis muscle spasm.

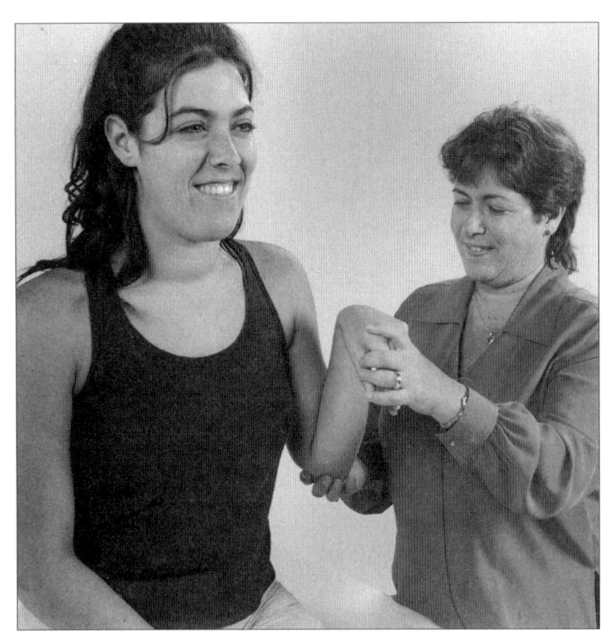

Medial Epicondyle (MEP)

Upper Extremity Dysfunction

EVALUATE

Limitation of Motion: Elbow supination.

TENDER POINT

High on medial epicondyle.

TREATMENT

- Supine or sitting.
- Ipsilateral elbow flexion with overpressure.
- Ipsilateral wrist flexion with overpressure.
- Ipsilateral forearm pronation to end of range.
- **Synergic Pattern Release**

Palmer Side Wrist Dysfunction

Wrist and Hand Dysfunction

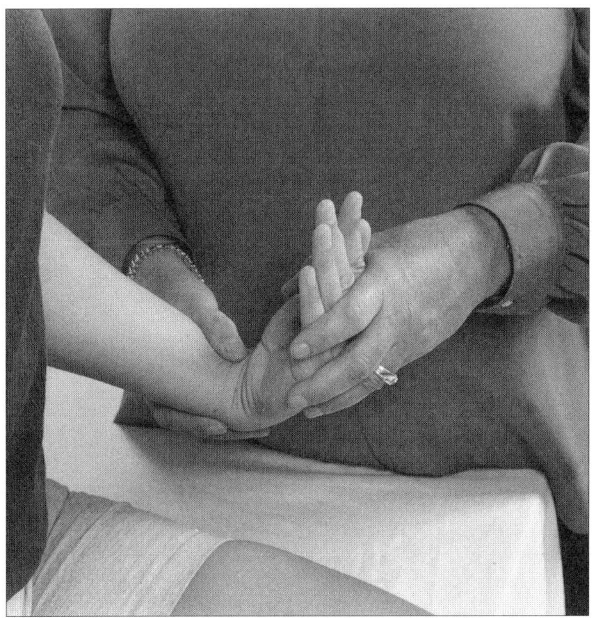

EVALUATE

Limitation of Motion: Wrist extension.

TENDER POINT

Palmer side of wrist.

TREATMENT

- Sitting or supine.
- Wrist flexion with overpressure.
- Sidebending towards the Tender Point.
- Fine tune with pronation and supination.
- **Synergic Pattern Release**

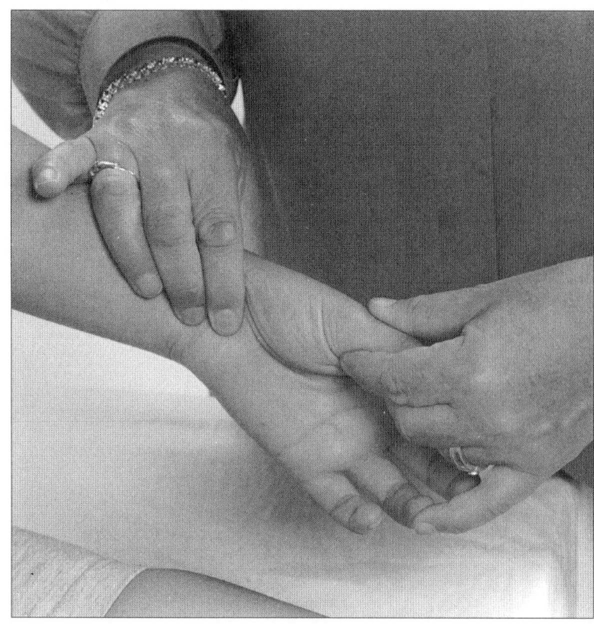

First Carpometacarpal Joint

Wrist and Hand Dysfunction

EVALUATE

Limitation of Motion: Thumb abduction and extension.

TENDER POINT

Deep at the medial aspect of the proximal head of first metacarpal.

TREATMENT

- Supine or sitting.
- Internal rotation of thumb with overpressure.
- Abduction of the thumb.
- Flexion of the thumb.
- **Synergic Pattern Release**

INTEGRATIVE MANUAL THERAPY

This is the technique to reduce a subluxed thumb, the type from trauma, for example a common ski injury. Excellent for De Quervains and tendinitis, this technique restores articular balance for the first carpal-metacarpal joint.

Interosseous Joints

Wrist and Hand Dysfunction

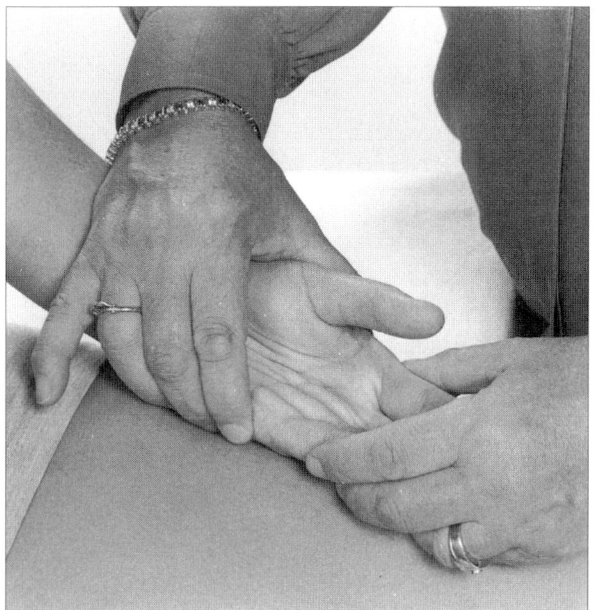

EVALUATE

Limitation of Motion: Finger extension and abduction.

TENDER POINT

Palmar side of hand, on the sides of the shafts of the metacarpal bones, medial and lateral (symptom: flexed interphalangeal joint).

TREATMENT

- Sitting or supine.
- Flexion with overpressure at the metacarpophalangeal joint.
- Fine tune: side pressure on the finger toward the affected palmar interosseous muscle.

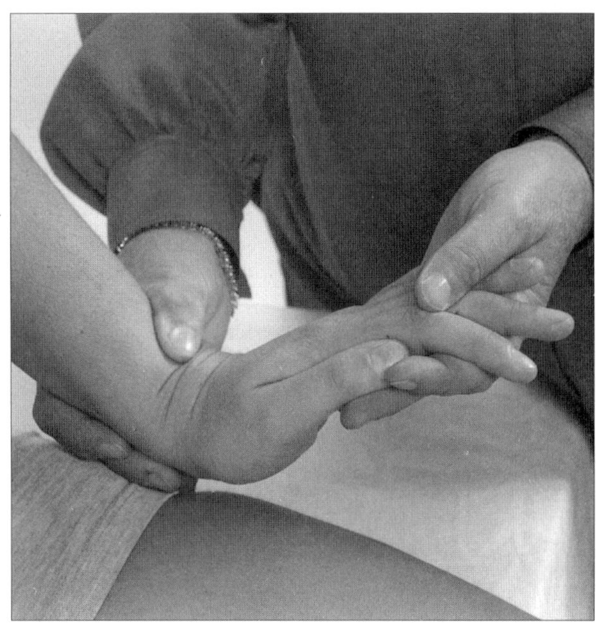

Dorsal Wrist

Wrist and Hand Dysfunction

EVALUATE

Limitation of Motion: Wrist flexion and mobility.

TENDER POINT

Dorsal aspect of wrist.

TREATMENT

- Supine or sitting.
- Extend wrist with overpressure.
- Fine tune with pronation or supination and side bending towards the side of the Tender Point.

CHAPTER 12

MYOFASCIAL RELEASE

A 3-PLANAR FASCIAL FULCRUM APPROACH TO CORRECT SOFT TISSUE AND JOINT DYSFUNCTION WITH DE-FACILITATED FASCIAL RELEASE

This concept was developed at Regional Physical Therapy. The technique is invaluable to improve arthrokinematics with a 3-Planar Fascial Fulcrum Release, (Weiselfish) Giammatteo, to address capsular and ligamentous tension and instability.

The Process of De-Facilitated Fascial Release with Strain and Counterstrain

- Position the body for Strain and Counterstrain (use the techniques from Chapters 8 and 9).
- Maintain the position for 90 seconds (2 to 3 minutes for the neurologic patient).
- Focus on all tissue tension changes, movements, pulses, rhythms.
- While there are changes occurring, maintain the Strain and Counterstrain position with precisely the same forces, not allowing any physiologic movement to occur.
- Continue to maintain this position until all tissue tension changes have ceased completely.

The practitioner is maintaining a fixed point around which the tissue can unravel (Fascial Fulcrum Release). The unwinding of the fascial tissue that occurs secondary to the continuation of the Strain and Counterstrain technique will happen secondary to the de-facilitation of the spinal segments. This unwinding will not occur unless initiated with the Strain and Counterstrain.

Often, significant improvements in arthrokinematics occur after this approach, and posture will reflect these changes. Mobility and ranges of motion will be increased. Ligamentous instability responds well to this approach. After several Strain and Counterstrain techniques, the tissue is ready to respond in this manner.

De-Facilitated Fascial Release can be implemented with: (1) Strain and Counterstrain Technique, (2) Muscle Energy and 'Beyond' Technique, and (3) Myofascial Release.

Fascial Concepts

Tissues are the matrix of the body, composed of cellular elements and their derivatives. The cells may be held together by the adhesions of their surface membranes, or by protoplasmic connections; they may be scattered throughout an intercellular ground substance containing tissue fluid, fibrous elements, and organic material. A tissue is a collection of cellular and fibrous elements in which one unique type of cell or fiber predominates. The four primary body tissues include: epithelial tissue for protection, secretion, and absorption; muscular tissue for contraction; nervous tissue for irritability and conductivity; connective tissue for support, nutrition, and defense.

The largest component of the human body, connective tissue, forms a continuous, contiguous system throughout the body. The connective tissue system includes all the components of the mesenchyme: ground substance, elastin, collagen, muscle, bone, cartilage, and adipose tissue. The various components of connective tissue are not distinct, but present many transitional forms. These components of connective tissue are characterized by large amounts of intercellular material. The consistency of the connective tissue is dependent upon the relative amount and proportion of collagenous and elastic fibers. Some areas of the body have thin, delicate reticulum, and other areas present tough fibrous sheets. The connective tissue is a highly specialized and complex tissue. The connective tissue contains and comprises blood vessels and lymphatic vessels in order to implement the functions of nutrition, defense, and repair. The cells and fibers dispersed throughout the connective tissue system are embedded in a matrix of semifluid gelatinous substance. Connective tissue can be grouped as follows:

Connective Tissue Proper

- Loose connective tissue (areolar). This tissue contains spaces of fluid, and is involved in cellular metabolism. Intercellular substances include: (a) collagenous or white fibers: collagen fibers are parallel fibers bound together in bundles giving it tensile strength; (b) elastic or yellow fibers: elastin contributes to the elasticity; (c) reticular fibers: the delicate collagenous fibers function to support cells.
- Dense connective tissues.
- Regular connective tissues: tendon, fibrous membranes, lamellated connective tissue.

Special Connective Tissue

- Mucous
- Elastin: fibers running singly, branching freely, and anastomosing with each other
- Reticular
- Adipose
- Pigmented

Amorphous

- Ground
- Cement

Cartilage

Bone

Blood and Lymph

Connective tissue has various functions. This system provides the supporting matrix for highly specialized organs and structures. It provides pathways for nerves, blood vessels, and lymphatic vessels, by organization of fascial planes. The connective tissue facilitates movement between the adjacent structures. It forms bursal sacs to minimize the effects of pressure and friction in the body. Connective tissue creates restraining mechanisms in the form of bands, pulleys, and ligaments. It aids in promoting circulation of veins and lymphatics by providing sheaths. It furnishes the sites for muscle attachments. It forms spaces for storage of fat to conserve body heat. It has fibroblastic activity in order to repair tissue injury by forming scar tissue. Connective tissue contains histocytes, which is a connective tissue cell that participates in phagocytic activity to defend against bacteria. The connective tissue synthesizes antibodies to neutralize antigens by its plasma cells, which are another connective tissue cell. It contains tissue fluids to participate in tissue nutrition.

Fascia is specialized connective tissue. Fascia envelops muscle fibers, and acts as a lubricant to permit freedom of movement of adjacent muscle groups. Tendons are bundles of heavy collagen fibers running parallel to one another. Tendons connect muscles to bone and can sustain enormous tension. Ligaments are similar to tendons, but the collagen fibers are not arranged as regularly and may contain some elastic fibers. Ligaments usually connect bone to bone. Cartilage is a fibrous connective tissue with a firm matrix. The cells are called chondrocytes. Hyaline, fibrocartilage, and elastin are specific types of cartilage. Muscle has often been considered a specialized form of connective tissue, the smooth and voluntary striated muscles. Bone and cartilage have been considered modified forms of collagen. Bone is harder connective tissue, in which large amounts of calcium comprise a solid matrix of fibrous connective tissue.

Fascia is a tough connective tissue that

spreads in a functional three-dimensional web from the head to the toe. Fascia gives the body form; if all other tissues and structures were removed from the body, the body would retain its shape. This is because every muscle, bone, organ, nerve, and vessel is wrapped in fascia. The fascia separates, supports, binds, connects, and defends everything. The fascia extends to form muscular attachments, to support membranes, to provide intermuscular septa, to give visceral ligamentous attachments, and to invest sheaths for blood vessels and nerves. The connective tissue found in the interstitial tissues of the viscera forms the membranes through which the osmotic processes of nutrition and elimination take place. The pressure and tissue tension provided by the fascia have a marked influence upon the osmotic exchange of fluid. The fascia affects the delivery of the metabolites into the filtering capillaries. The fascia affects the osmotic balance which exists between the circulatory fluids and the tissue fluids, which preserves physiologic balance. Functionally, the fascia can be separated into layers: the superficial fascia, which adheres to the undersurface of the skin and the deep fascia, which envelopes and separates muscles, surrounds and separates internal organs, and contributes to the contour and function of the body.

Specializations of the deep fascia include the peritoneum, the pericardium, and the pleura. Subserous fascia is the loose areolar tissue which envelops the viscera. This fascia provides friction-free movement between the organs. The deepest fascia is the dura mater. All these tissues are connected continuously and contiguously.

The intercranial structures are connected through the foramina at the base of the skull. Within the chest cavity, the pericardium extends upwards to become continuous with the pre-tracheal layer of the deep cervical fascia, and below is attached to the diaphragm. The heart is suspended in the chest by the attachments of the pericardium and related fascia. The pericardium is connected with the mediastinal pleura. The mediastinal fascia connects the bifurcation of the trachea, the descending aorta and the esophagus. The abdominal fascia includes the mesentery, the omentum, and numerous ligaments which provide support for the abdominal viscera. The omentum consists of a fold of the peritoneum, and is attached to various portions of the abdominal wall and forms ligaments to maintain the position of solid viscera. The cervical visceral fascia extends from the base of the skull to the mediastinum, forming compartments for the esophagus, the trachea, and the carotid vessels, and providing support for the pharynx, larynx, and thyroid gland.

The connective tissue is comprised of collagen, elastin, and the polysaccharide gel complex, the ground substance. Collagen is a protein of three polypeptide chains which provide strength to this fascial tissue. Elastin is a protein which is rubber-like and absorbs tensile forces. Together, the elastin and collagen combine to form an elastocollagenous complex. The polysaccharide gel fills a space between the fibers. The major components are hyaluronic acid and proteoglycans. Hyaluronic acid is viscous, and provides lubrication for the collagen, elastin, and muscle fibers allowing for friction-free movement. Proteoglycans are peptide chains which contribute to the gel of the ground substance, which is hydrophilic and thereby rich in water content.

Manual Therapy and Fascial/Myofascial Dysfunction

Neuromusculoskeletal dysfunction causes postural dysfunction. Postural dysfunction produces fascial tensions. The traction produced by postural dysfunction upon the sensory nerve elements within the connective tissue system may produce pain.

As a manual practitioner develops the specialized sense of touch necessary for diagnosis of tissue disorders, differential diagnosis is facilitated. Education of tactile senses can determine if tissue is tense, relaxed, or altered due to imbalance of tissue chemistry. The development of palpation skills is essential for diagnosing fascial dysfunction.

Fascial dysfunction can contribute to changes in health: local, regional, and total body. Ligamentous tension alterations are important in joint lesion pathology. Stretching of ligaments can result in hypermobility of joints. Dislocations of bone, whether mild with imbalance of the articular surfaces, or severe, will result in tendon tension. This tendon tension is transmitted to muscle fibers, which produces compensatory hypertonicity and muscle contractions.

Immobilization may result in fascial dysfunction. Research has provided evidence that long periods of immobilization produces muscle atrophy, joint stiffness, ulceration of joint cartilage, osteoarthritis, skin necrosis, infection, tendocutaneous adhesion, thrombophlebitis, and varying degrees of contracture. Research has provided evidence that synovial fluid post immobilization has excessive connective tissue deposition in the joint and joint recesses. After a time, the excessive fibrous connective tissue deposits form mature scar and create intra-articular adhesions. Post immobilization, matrix changes have been reported in ligament, capsule, tendon, and fascia. Research has also provided evidence that functional loading can cause regeneration of tendons. Enwemeka performed research which showed that controlled passive mobilization promotes gliding and accelerates the rate of healing of tendons. With the mobilization, reports of water loss, increased synthesis of new collagen, and an increase in the cross-links between collagen fibers have been presented. The excessive and abnormal cross-link formation between fibers contributes to joint restriction.

Fascial Release Techniques can be Direct or Indirect Techniques.

Direct Techniques

The tissues are moved to the barrier on three planes. The tissues are loaded in the direction of the least mobility. A relaxation in the tissue tension will result from the treatment, and heat will be released in the tissues. *The author and colleagues emphasize the point that indirect techniques cause less body resistance and provide more effective and efficient results.*

Indirect Techniques

The tissues/joints are moved away from the barrier on three planes, into the direction of the most mobility. The tissues/joints are unloaded. A relaxation in the tissue tension will result from the treatment, and heat will be released from the tissues.

Tissue Release

The therapist monitors tissue tension during manual therapy techniques. When the tissue tension changes, softens and relaxes, this is a tissue release. These releases occur during a treatment technique.

This decrease in tissue tension during manual therapy has been attributed to several factors. One factor is the decrease in gamma gain and efferent gain from the central nervous system, resulting in a relaxation and elongation of muscle fibers. Another factor is the change of elastic resistance to viscous compliance due to morphologic changes. There is an apparent relaxation of these elastic fibers. Tissue tension release occurs simultaneously with a perception of increased fluid throughout the tissues, and a sense of increased energy throughout those tissues treated. During the treatment technique, heat is emanated from those body tissues, there is a sensation of movement, filling of space, and often a therapeutic pulse.

This *therapeutic pulse* occurs frequently during manual therapy techniques. The amplitude or force of this therapeutic pulse increases during the treatment technique and subsides as the correction of the neuromusculoskeletal tissue is completed.

Fascial Fulcrum Techniques

There are two generic Fascial Fulcrum techniques:

- Soft Tissue Fulcrum Myofascial Release
- Articular Fulcrum Fascial Release

Application

These techniques can be performed mechanically with excellent results. Development of palpation skills will enhance these results.

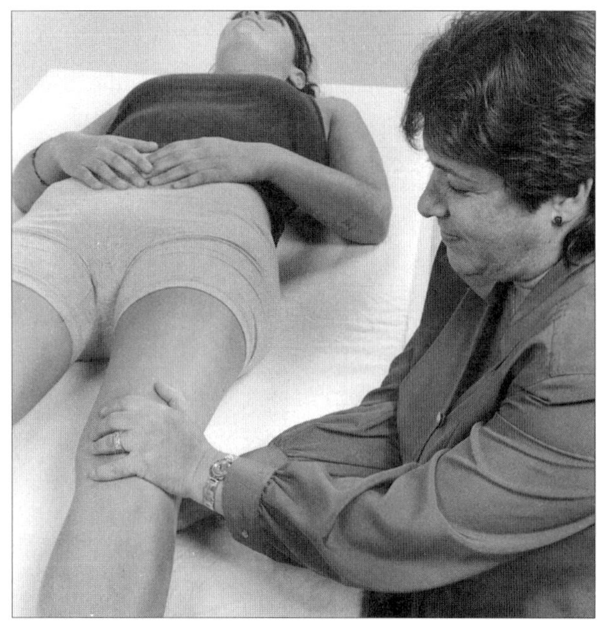

Soft Tissue Myofascial Release Technique

Soft Tissue Myofascial Release techniques can be performed where positive myofascial mapping, decreased fascial glide, static postural dysfunction, and dynamic limitations in motion indicate positive findings of dysfunction.

Example #1:
Soft Tissue Myofascial Release of the Knee

INDICATION

Pain, postural dysfunction, limitations in knee motions.

POSITION

Supine. One hand of the therapist is underneath the knee joint. The fingers are spread apart, contacting as much tissue and structure as possible. The second hand of the therapist rests above the knee joint. The fingers are spread apart, contacting as many tissues and structures as possible.

TREATMENT

1. *Compress* the knee with both hands, squeezing gently, imaging a soap bubble between the hands. Don't burst the soap bubble! Maintain the gentle compression.
2. *First Plane*: The anterior hand moves cephalad while the posterior hand moves caudad, distorting the soap bubble. The hands return to neutral and reverse directions: the anterior hand moves the tissue caudad, while the posterior hand moves the tissue cephalad. Consider: Which direction (cephalad/caudad or caudad/cephalad) was the mobility greatest, with least resistance? Move the hands in the "indirect" direction of ease. Keep hands in that new position.
3. *Second Plane*: Now add, or "stack" the second plane movements. Do not return the hands or the tissues to neutral. Move the

tissues under the anterior hand medially, while the posterior hand moves the tissue laterally. Return the tissues to neutral, and compare the ease of tissue mobility when the anterior hand moves the tissue laterally while the posterior hand moves the tissue medially. Consider: Which directions (medial/lateral or lateral/medial) were the most mobile, the easiest, the least restricted? Return the tissues to that position. Maintain these directions of forces on the tissues, as well as those forces from the first plane.

4. *Third Plane*: Now add, or "stack" the third plane. Do not return the tissues to neutral; they are displaced from neutral on two planes now. Move the tissues with the anterior hand in a clockwise direction, while the posterior hand moves the tissues in a counterclockwise direction. Then return the tissues to neutral on this plane; compare the opposite tissue distortion pattern. Move the tissues counterclockwise with the anterior hand, while the posterior hand moves the tissues clockwise. Compare the two different tissue distortion patterns (clockwise/counterclockwise or counterclockwise/clockwise): Which was the indirect pattern with the greatest mobility? Return the tissues in that direction of distortion. Now there are three directions of forces from each hand onto the tissues; each hand is displacing the tissues on three planes.
5. *The Fulcrum*: Each hand exerted four different directions of forces mechanically to distort the tissue between the hands. The directions of force were:
   - compression
   - superior or inferior
   - medial or lateral
   - clockwise or counterclockwise (medial rotation or lateral rotation)
6. Each hand will now maintain all four directions of forces, maintaining a fulcrum for the tissue unwinding, throughout the duration of the technique. This fulcrum will create energy which will be transmitted into the body.
7. *Maintaining the Fulcrum*: As the tissue unwinds, and movement occurs in the body's internal environment, there is a temptation to move the hands and release the fulcrum. Resist the temptation. The therapist and patient may perceive heat, paresthesia, anaesthesia, vibration, fatigue, electricity, cold, perspiration, pain, circulatory changes, breathing changes, sympathetic skin erythemia or blanching, and more. Do not release the fulcrum; at the end of the technique the signs and symptoms will subside. The technique is complete when all movement, signs, symptoms, and perceptions have ceased.

RESULT:

Improved postural symmetry, decreased pain, increased knee movements.

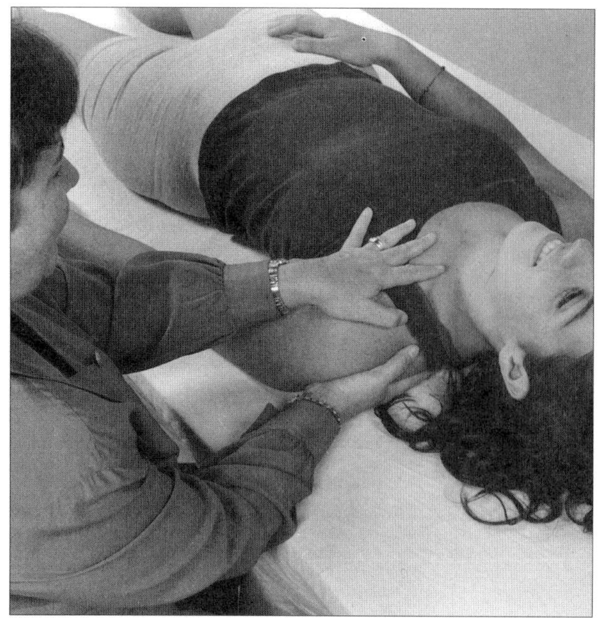

Example #2: Soft Tissue Myofascial Release of the Shoulder Girdle and Clavipectoral Fascia

INDICATION

Pain, postural dysfunction, limitations in shoulder motions.

POSITION

Supine or sitting. One hand of the therapist rests on the anterior clavipectoral region. The fingers are spread apart, contacting as much tissue and structure as possible. The second hand of the therapist is underneath the scapula and posterior glenoid. The fingers are spread apart, contacting as many tissues and structures as possible.

TREATMENT

1. *Compress* the clavipectoral region with both hands, squeezing gently, imaging a soap bubble between the hands. Don't burst the soap bubble! Maintain the gentle compression.
2. *First Plane*: The anterior hand moves cephalad while the posterior hand moves caudal, distorting the soap bubble. The hands return to neutral and reverse directions: the anterior hand moves the tissue caudal, while the posterior hand moves the tissue cephalad. Consider: Which direction (cephalad/caudad or caudad/ cephalad) was the mobility greatest, with least resistance? The hands move the tissues in the "indirect" direction of ease, the most mobile direction. Keep hands in that new position, maintaining those directions of forces on the tissues.
3. *Second Plane*: Now add, or "stack" the second plane movements. Do not return the hands or the tissues to neutral. Move the tissues under the anterior hand medially,

while the posterior hand moves the tissue laterally. Return the tissues to neutral, and compare the ease of tissue mobility when the anterior hand moves the tissue laterally while the posterior hand moves the tissue medially. Consider: Which directions (medial/lateral or lateral/medial) were the most mobile, the easiest, the least restricted? Return the tissues to that position. Maintain these directions of forces on the tissues, as well as those forces from the first plane.

4. *Third Plane*: Now add, or "stack" the third plane. Do not return the tissues to neutral; they are displaced from neutral on two planes now. Move the tissues with the anterior hand in a clockwise direction, while the posterior hand moves the tissues in a counterclockwise direction. Then return the tissues to neutral on this plane; compare the opposite tissue distortion pattern. Move the tissues counterclockwise with the anterior hand, while the posterior hand moves the tissues clockwise. Compare the two different tissue distortion patterns (clockwise/counterclockwise or counterclockwise/clockwise): Which was the indirect pattern with the greatest mobility? Return the tissues in that direction of distortion. Now there are three directions of forces from each hand onto the tissues; each hand is displacing the tissues on three planes.
5. *The Fulcrum*: Each hand exerted four different directions of forces mechanically to distort the tissue between the hands. The directions of force were:
   - compression
   - superior/inferior
   - medial/lateral
   - clockwise/counterclockwise (medial rotation or lateral rotation)

   Each hand will now maintain all four directions of force, maintaining a fulcrum for the tissue unwinding, throughout the duration of the technique. This fulcrum will create energy which will be transmitted into the body.
6. *Maintaining the Fulcrum*: As the tissue unwinds, and movement occurs in the body's internal environment, there is a temptation to move the hands and release the fulcrum. Resist the temptation. The therapist and patient may perceive heat, paresthesia, anaesthesia, vibration, fatigue, electricity, cold, perspiration, pain, circulatory changes, breathing changes, sympathetic skin erythemia or blanching, and more. Do not release the fulcrum; at the end of the technique the signs and symptoms will subside. The technique is complete when all movement, signs, symptoms, and perceptions have ceased.

RESULT

Improved postural symmetry (decreased protraction) and increased horizontal abduction.

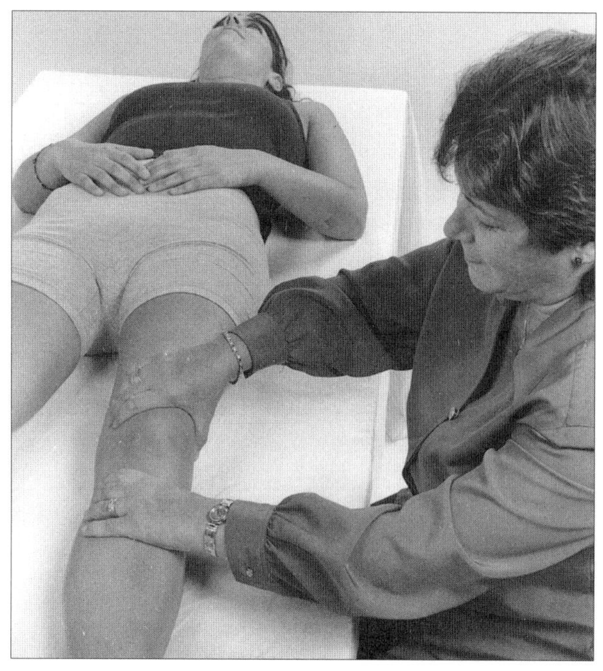

Articular Fascial Release Technique

Articular Fascial Release techniques can be performed where positive myofascial mapping is palpated over any joint. Articular Fascial Release is indicated for any musculoskeletal fascial dysfunction involving the joint capsule, ligaments, tendons and other joint-related tissues.

Example #1: Articular Fascial Release of the Knee Joint

INDICATION

Localized postural dysfunction at the knee joint; lateral shear of the proximal tibial head on the distal femoral head.

POSITION

Supine. One hand of the therapist grips the distal femur head The second hand grips the proximal tibial head. *Do not distract or approximate the joint surfaces.*

TREATMENT

1. *First Plane*: The superior hand on the femur lifts the femoral head anterior, while the inferior hand on the tibia pulls the tibial head posterior. Then return to neutral and reverse the directions. The superior hand pushes the femur posterior, while the inferior hand pushes the tibial head anterior. Compare: Which direction (anterior/posterior or posterior/anterior) was the most mobile? Return the joint surfaces to that position of greatest mobility. Maintain the position of the articular surfaces on this plane.
2. *Second Plane*: Now add, or "stack" the second plane movements. The superior hand holding the femoral head can push the femur lateral, while the inferior hand holding the tibia can push the tibial head medial. Then return to neutral and reverse the directions of the articular surfaces. The

superior hand now pushes the femur medial, while the inferior hand pushes the tibia lateral. Compare the directions (medial/lateral or lateral/medial). Move the joint surfaces in the indirect directions of ease. Maintain the articular surfaces in this new position.

3. *Third Plane*: Now add, or "stack" the third plane movements. The superior hand gripping the femur can rotate the femoral head externally, while the inferior hand gripping the tibia rotates the tibial surface internally. Then return to neutral, and reverse the directions. The superior hand can push the femoral head into internal rotation, while the inferior hand moves the tibia into external rotation. Compare the directions (external/internal rotations or internal/external rotations). Move the articular surfaces on this plane in the indirect direction of greatest mobility, least resistance. Maintain the positions of the articular surfaces on this plane.
4. *The Fulcrum*: Each hand has exerted three different directions of mechanical forces to position the articular surfaces in opposite directions on three planes. Each hand will now maintain all three directions of forces, maintaining a fulcrum for the unwinding tissue of the joint capsule and ligaments throughout the duration of the technique.
5. *Maintaining the Fulcrum*: As the tissue unwinds, and sensations of extra-articular and intra-articular movement are perceived, there is a temptation to move the hands and release the fulcrum. Resist the temptation to release the fulcrum. Maintain the fulcrum until all movement, all signs, all symptoms and all perceptions have ceased.

RESULT

Improved articular balance. Normal neutral balance of femoral head and tibial head; increased joint mobility; increased ranges of knee motions.

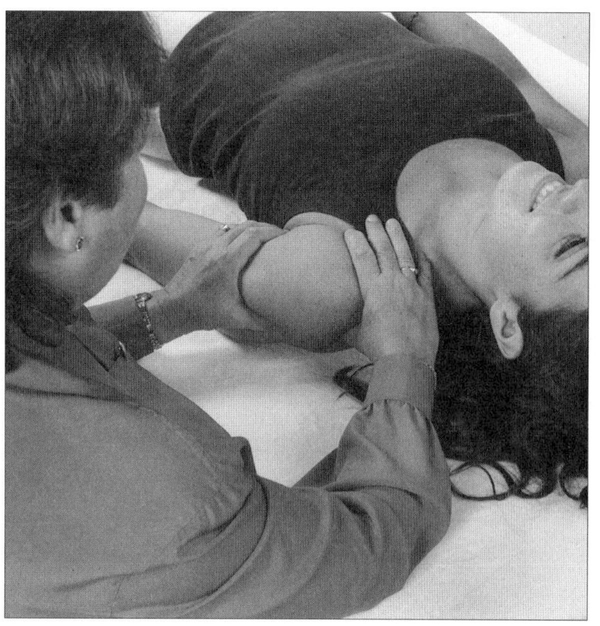

Example #2: Treatment of the Glenohumeral Joint with Articular Fascial Release

INDICATION

Static postural dysfunction: For example, anterior shear of the humeral head in the glenoid fossa.

Dynamic postural dysfunction: Limitation in some end ranges of shoulder motions, with hypomobility of accessory movements evident on mobility testing.

POSITION

Supine or sitting. One hand of the therapist grips the shoulder girdle to control the position of the glenoid fossa. The second hand grips the upper arm to control the position of the humeral head. *Do not distract or approximate the joint surfaces.*

TREATMENT

1. *First Plane*: The superior hand on the shoulder girdle lifts the glenoid fossa cephalad, while the inferior hand on the upper arm pulls the humeral head caudad. Then return the joint surfaces to neutral, and reverse the directions of the articular surfaces. The superior hand pushes the glenoid fossa caudad, while the inferior hand pushes the humeral head cephalad. Compare: Which direction (cephalad/caudad or caudad/cephalad) was the most mobile, the least restricted and the least inhibited? Return the joint surfaces to that position of greatest mobility. Maintain the position of the articular surfaces on this plane.
2. *Second Plane*: Now add, or "stack" the second plane movements. The superior hand holding the shoulder girdle can push the glenoid fossa anteriorly, while the inferior hand holding the upper arm can

push the humeral head posteriorly. Then return the joint surfaces to neutral and reverse the directions of the articular surfaces. The superior hand now pushes the glenoid fossa posteriorly, while the inferior hand pushes the humeral head anteriorly. Compare the directions (anterior/posterior or posterior/anterior). Move the joint surfaces in the indirect directions of ease. Maintain the articular surfaces in this new position. Now each articular surface is displaced in different directions.

3. *Third Plane*: Now add, or "stack" the third plane movements. The superior hand gripping the shoulder girdle can rotate the glenoid fossa externally, while the inferior hand gripping the upper arm rotates the humeral head internally. Then return the joint surfaces to neutral, and reverse the directions. The superior hand can push the glenoid fossa into internal rotation, while the inferior hand moves the humeral head into external rotation. Compare the directions (external/internal rotations or internal/external rotations). Move the articular surfaces on this plane in the indirect direction of greatest mobility, least resistance. Maintain the positions of the articular surfaces on this plane. Now the three directions of forces exerted to displace each articular surface is maintained.
4. *The Fulcrum*: Each hand has exerted three different directions of forces to mechanically move and position the articular surfaces in opposite directions on three planes. Each hand will now maintain all three directions of forces, maintaining a fulcrum for the unwinding tissue of the joint capsule and ligaments throughout the duration of the technique.
5. *Maintaining the Fulcrum*: As the tissue unwinds, and sensations of extra-articular and intra-articular movement are perceived, there is a temptation to move the hands and release the fulcrum. Resist the temptation to release the fulcrum. Maintain the fulcrum until all movement, all signs, all symptoms and all perceptions have ceased.

RESULT

Improved articular balance. Normal neutral balance of humeral head within the glenoid fossa; increased joint mobility; increased ranges of shoulder motions.

CHAPTER 13

TENDON RELEASE THERAPY

FOR TREATMENT OF TENDON TISSUE TENSION WITH ADVANCED STRAIN AND COUNTERSTRAIN

The tendons are innervated by the autonomic nervous system, because functionally, they respond in a similar manner to smooth muscles. There is a passive contractile function, which is required for the stretch reflex of the proprioceptors, such as the Golgi apparatus. The contractile tissues are longitudinal along the length of the tendon. When there is hypertonicity of a tendon, it presents as a rigidity of the tendon. There is a reduced capacity of elongation and contraction of the tendon fibers.

Duration of treatment of tendons with Advanced Strain and Counterstrain is 1 minute because all innervated muscles require 1 minute for release of hypertonicity, as compared to 90 seconds required for release of the voluntary nervous system innervated muscles. This approach was developed by Giammatteo and (Weiselfish) Giammatteo, incorporated into their text on Advanced Strain and Counterstrain Technique. The process of De-Facilitated Fascial Release works well with tendon hypertonicity.

Tendons of voluntary striated muscles are treated in a relatively simple manner with Advanced Strain and Counterstrain Technique, with excellent results. There may remain fascial restrictions of the tendon, which may still require fascial release. The tendon responds well to De-Facilitated Fascial Release.

Indications

There are essentially no contra-indications for Tendon Release Therapy when performed in this manner, unless there is a total rupture of the tendon. When there is a total rupture of the tendon, the technique will not be effective.

If there is a tear or rupture of the tendon, but there is a correction performed (surgical), the technique can be performed. Although not 100 percent effective, the technique will give some results in decreased hypertonicity and rigidity of the tendon if the Tendon Release Therapy is performed immediately after surgery. There will be a facilitated healing of the tendinous injury.

Tendon Release Therapy is best performed after Strain and Counterstrain is performed to the muscle of the tendon. Often there is no remaining hypertonicity of the muscle, only of the tendon. In that case, Tendon Release Therapy can be performed without Strain and Counterstrain to the muscle.

After Tendon Release Therapy is performed, there may be some residual fascial dysfunction of the connective tissue of the tendon. This occurs most often when there are tears and scarring of the tendon. After the Tendon Release Therapy, a 3-Planar Fascial Fulcrum Release Technique (Myofascial Release, (Weiselfish) Giammatteo) can be performed for optimal results. The Advanced Strain and Counterstrain for the tendon (Tendon Release Therapy) affects the hypertonicity of the tendon, resulting in a softening of the tendon and a decrease in the rigid presentation of that tendon. When De-Facilitated Fascial Release is performed immediately after the Tendon Release Therapy, often the fascial dysfunction is corrected. When the scarring of the tendon (the fibrosis) is severe, there is often a need to perform the fascial release after the Tendon Release Therapy.

Sequence of Integrative Manual Therapy for Tendons

1. Muscle Energy and 'Beyond' Technique for extremity joints.
2. Strain and Counterstrain for the muscle (of the involved tendon).
3. De-Facilitated Fascial Release for the muscle (of the involved tendon).
4. Tendon Release Therapy (Advanced Strain and Counterstrain).
5. De-Facilitated Fascial Release for the tendon.
6. Myofascial Release (3-Planar Fascial Fulcrum) Tendon Technique.

Treatment

1. Place the index finger (or the index finger plus the third finger) pad of the distal phalanx of the caudal hand over the place of insertion of the inferior end of the tendon.
2. Place the index finger (or the index finger plus third finger) pad of the distal phalanx of the superior hand over the musculotendinous interface of the muscle/tendon, at the superior aspect of the tendon.
3. Push on the tendon tissue with both hands (fingers) with a 1 pound force perpendicular onto the bone.
4. Then compress the superior aspects and inferior aspects of the tendon together with a 1 pound force, bringing the proximal and distal ends of the tendon closer together.
5. Maintain these (4) compressive forces for one minute for the Advanced Strain and Counterstrain.
6. If fascial unwinding is perceived, maintain the (4) compressive forces during a De-Facilitated Fascial Release.

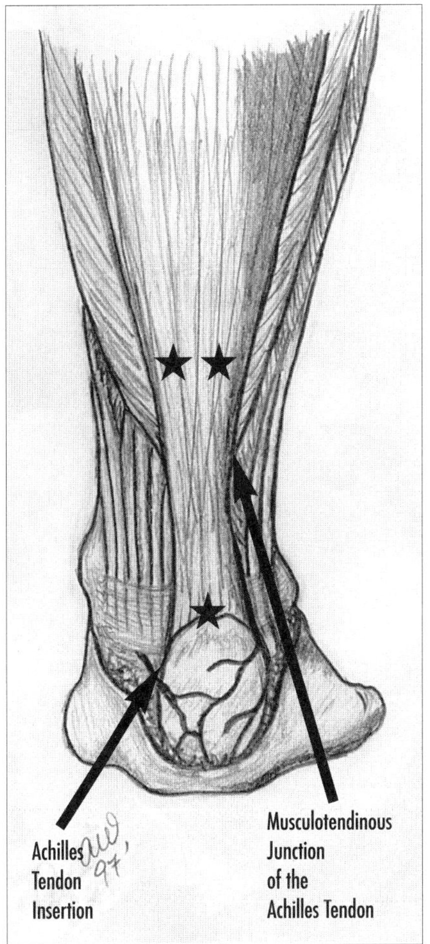

Figure 17. To perform Tendon Release Therapy, press on the musculotendinous junction and on the insertion of the Achilles tendon. Then shorten the fibers.

Indications for Tendon Release Therapy

Typical tendons which respond well with Tendon Release Therapy:

- Achilles tendon
- Medial and lateral hamstrings tendons
- Quadriceps tendon
- Tibialis anterior tendon
- Tibialis posterior tendon
- Extensor tendons of the foot and toes
- Flexor tendons of the foot and toes
- Abductor hallucis
- Adductor tendons of the hip
- Rotator cuff tendons: supraspinatus, infraspinatus, subscapularis
- Latissimus dorsi
- Biceps tendons (short head and long head)
- Triceps tendon
- Coracobrachialis tendon
- Brachioradialis tendon
- Wrist flexor tendons
- Wrist extensor tendons
- Finger flexor tendons
- Finger extensor tendons
- Abductor pollicis tendon
- Flexor pollicis tendon

Common disorders which respond well to Tendon Release Therapy:

- Tendinitis
- Hypertonicity (protective muscle spasm and spasticity)
- Muscular dystrophies
- Hypotonias
- Fibromyalgias
- Tenosynovitis
- Tears and ruptures of tendons
- De Quervain-like syndromes
- Hallux valgus-like syndromes
- Tendon calcifications, such as calcification of supraspinatus tendon and bicipital tendon calcification

Example: Treatment of Achilles Tendon with Tendon Release Therapy

TENDER POINT

At the insertion of the Achilles tendon.

TREATMENT

1. Prone. A small towel roll is placed under the ankle, or the foot is off the edge of the bed, so that the foot and ankle are not in forced plantar flexion.
2. Place the index finger (or index finger plus the third finger) pad of the distal phalanx of the caudal hand over the place of insertion of the Achilles tendon at the calcaneus.
3. Place the index finger (or index finger plus third finger) pad of the distal phalanx of the superior hand over the musculotendinous interface of the gastrocnemius muscle with the Achilles tendon, at the superior aspect of the tendon.
4. Push the tissue with a 1 pound force perpendicular into the tibia. Then compress the superior aspect and inferior aspect of the tendon together with about a 1 pound force, bringing the two ends of the tendon closer together. Maintain these compressive forces.

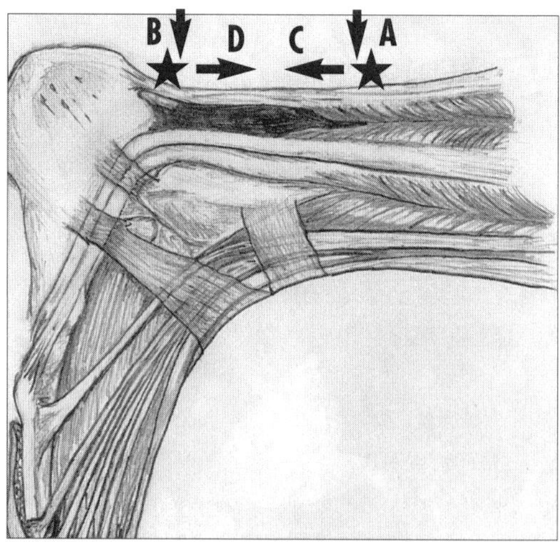

Figure 18. Tendon Release Therapy for the Achilles tendon. *Step 1:* Compress **A** and **B** posterior to anterior. *Step 2:* Shorten the length of the tendon (**C** and **D**). Maintain for 90 seconds.

CHAPTER 14

LIGAMENTS: A TENSILE FORCE GUIDANCE SYSTEM

TREATMENT WITH LIGAMENT FIBER THERAPY

The body has a system of ligaments which responds with tension/force that is partially due to the energies within the intra-articular space. Those energies which are within the intra-articular space are particle and wave presentations that can be defined in quantum physics terms. These energies present three-dimensional forces that affect the tension of the ligaments and these ligaments react to this tension with a force that is longitudinal as well as horizontal.

Ligaments are connective tissue that have elastin, collagen, ground substance, as well as cells and other crystallized entities. The elastin and collagen respond in manners similar to the binding/supporting functions of fascial tissues such as the iliotibial band. The crystallized cells are apparently similar to the cells found in bone, which have an electrophysiologic and electromagnetic component which can respond for guidance. The function of the longitudinal force of ligaments is direction. The function of the horizontal force of ligaments is coordination, which affects balance.

There are lines of tension within the body from ligament to ligament. Essentially all ligaments in the body have lines of tension with other ligaments. These lines of tension are the energy waves which direct body parts during action, and which coordinate body parts during activity and movement. These lines of tension can be accessed by stretching ligaments. Each ligament is pulled in a longitudinal manner like a string; this string is between the two ligaments that are being pulled in that longitudinal manner. Direct longitudinal stretch with two ligaments at the same time will access this line of tension. In conditions of dysfunction, the line of tension may be compromised. A longitudinal stretch on both ligaments will access the lines of tension, and will alleviate the compromise of the line of tension between these two ligaments. The result will be improved direction of motion from the body part guided by this line of tension, which probably responds to electrophysiologic internal signals and electromagnetic external forces.

The horizontal force of the ligament is more difficult to address. Within the ligaments are horizontal forces that are the coordinating forces of that body part during action and movement. The horizontal force of the ligament coordinates the neighboring body parts that the ligament is attached to, so that the body parts which are attached will move in better relationship, one with the other. In order to access this horizontal force within the ligament for improved coordination, there is a technique that can induce wave-like formation of the force.

If the hand is placed on the ligament while the joint is moving, the hand can respond to this horizontal force with intention to align this wave-like force in a horizontal manner. This technique can be performed during sagittal plane movements (flexion and extension), during coronal plane movements (abduction and adduction, right and left side bending), and transverse plane movements (external and internal rotation). The hand rests on the ligament aligned in a horizontal manner in order to address the horizontal force within the ligament. From inner through outer range of each motion on each plane, this horizontal force can be aligned.

If there is a biomechanical problem within the joint affecting the 3-planar presentation of the energy within that joint in the intra-articular space, it may be premature to work on the ligament, especially in a horizontal alignment of forces. The longitudinal traction of the ligaments to address the line of tension to improve direction of that body part can often be addressed while addressing biomechanical dysfunction of the intra-articular space with Muscle Energy and 'Beyond' Technique. The horizontal force is less able to be corrected until there is a correction of biomechanical problems.

The movement for correction of the horizontal force can be in a weight bearing or non-weight bearing manner. The longitudinal traction on the ligament to access the line of tension and correct direction of the body part is best performed in a non-weight bearing manner.

Ligament Fiber Therapy (LFT)

Ligament Fiber Therapy was developed by (Weiselfish) Giammatteo to restore proliferation of ligament activity.

There are two stages to Ligament Fiber Therapy:
1. Horizontal Fiber Therapy (HFT)
2. Longitudinal Fiber Therapy (LFT)

Horizontal Fiber Therapy is usually performed before Longitudinal Fiber Therapy, in order to restore coordination of the joint, i.e., the co-joined activity of the two articular surfaces of the joint so that each joint surface is working correctly relative to the neighboring joint surface.

When to Use Ligament Fiber Therapy

The horizontal fibers of the ligaments are treated with a direct approach *after* therapy is performed, to treat local fascial restrictions. Usually, there is a need to perform a Soft Tissue Myofascial Release Technique, the 3-Planar Fascial Fulcrum Technique, at the joint (see Soft Tissue Myofascial Release Technique, Chapter 10). This technique is followed by an Articular Fascial Release Technique, the 3-Planar Fascial Fulcrum Technique, to the joint (see example: Articular Fascial Release of Knee Joint, Chapter 10). There are more specialized Myofascial Release techniques which are not presented in this book, for example:

- Ligament releases (Myofascial Release, (Weiselfish) Giammatteo) can be performed with the 3-Planar Fascial Fulcrum Approach to the ligaments surrounding the joint;
- Collateral ligament techniques (Myofascial Release, (Weiselfish) Giammatteo) are often appropriate.

Sequence of Integrative Manual Therapy for Ligaments

This protocol of Myofascial Release is often sufficient for mild and moderate joint pain and disability. When there are further problems with the joint, Ligament Fiber Therapy can be implemented.

1. First perform Strain and Counterstrain Technique to the muscles surrounding the treated joint (Chapters 8 and 9).
2. Then perform a 3-Planar Soft Tissue Myofascial Release Technique at the joint (Chapter 10).
3. Then perform a 3-Planar Articular Fascial Release Technique at the joint (Chapter 10).
4. Then perform Ligament Fiber Therapy.

Introducing Synchronizers

Synchronizers are reflex points. Use these reflex points to attain improved results. Do a technique, for example Ligament Fiber Therapy. Try to perform the technique with one hand; contact the reflex point with the second hand. Synchronizers were discovered by Lowen and (Weiselfish) Giammatteo, presented in courses of Biologic Analogs, presented by Therapeutic Horizons, which is a continuing education institute for advanced studies in manual therapy.

Stage One: Horizontal Fiber Therapy

Place the thenar or hypothenar eminence over the ligament. Place direct pressure in a perpendicular direction onto the ligament. Rotate the fibers of the ligament in a clockwise and a counterclockwise direction. Determine which direction, clockwise or counterclockwise, is more restricted. Maintaining the direct perpendicular pressure, rotate the ligament fibers in the restricted direction, to the end of amplitude without overpressure. Then torque the ligament in a sagittal plane, i.e., flexion and extension of the fibers. Stack this component, i.e., flex or extend (torque) the ligament in the sagittal plane direction which is more restricted. When these forces of direct pressure plus rotation plus torque are applied together, stretch the ligament fibers to achieve separation of the horizontal fibers.

SYNCHRONIZER FOR HFT

Situated 1 inch lateral to the umbilicus, then 2 inches caudal.

TREATMENT

1. Place the thenar or hypothenar eminence over the ligament.
2. Place direct pressure in a perpendicular direction onto the ligament.
3. Rotate the fibers of the ligament in a clockwise and a counterclockwise direction.
4. Determine which direction, clockwise or counterclockwise, is more restricted. Maintaining the direct perpendicular pressure, rotate the ligament fibers in the restricted direction, to the end of amplitude without overpressure.
5. Torque the ligament in a sagittal plane, i.e., flexion and extension of the fibers. Stack this component, i.e., flex or extend (torque) the ligament in the sagittal plane direction which is more restricted.
6. When these forces of direct pressure plus rotation plus torque are applied together, stretch the ligament fibers to achieve separation of the horizontal fibers.
7. Place the second hand on the synchronizer for Horizontal Fiber Therapy (1 inch lateral to the umbilicus and 2 inches caudal). Maintaining the fulcrum for the "Release": There will be a "Release" of the tissues, a change in tissue tension. Maintain the pressure and contact of both hands until the end of the "Release" when changes are no longer occurring in tissue tension.

Stage Two: Longitudinal Fiber Therapy (LFT)

Longitudinal Fiber Therapy is different from Horizontal Fiber Therapy. This is apparently because the longitudinal fibers of the ligaments are a "system" of ligamentous fibers, which contract and relax together, which respond to all changes in pressure and motion anywhere in the body as a "functional unit." The longitudinal fibers require a total body approach to therapy. These fibers are significant for many reasons.

Significance of Longitudinal Ligament Fibers

The ligament system appears to be a "guidance system" of the person. This means several important items:

- The longitudinal ligaments perform the "awareness function" for the distal bone of attachment: Is the distal bone moving in the correct direction according to brain function? Is the distal bone moving in the correct direction, according to the proximal bone of attachment?
- The longitudinal ligaments perform the "awareness function" of both the proximal and the distal bones of attachment: Is the person moving his/her body in accordance with higher consciousness? Is he/she "moving" on his/her Path? This aspect of the function of the longitudinal ligaments is presented at other educational forums, and will not be elaborated on in this text. This question of "ligament awareness" does appear to be significant whenever there is joint dysfunction affecting multiple joints: "Is the person 'being' in this life according to his/her unique Path?"

Treatment of longitudinal fibers of ligaments is a two-phase therapy. Phase One requires assessment and treatment of the individual ligament involved. Phase Two requires a total body approach.

Modification of Longitudinal Fiber Therapy (LFT) for the "Guidance System"

Longitudinal Fiber Therapy is modified in this text. LFT approach will be facilitated with Myofascial Mapping. When Myofascial Mapping is positive on a coronal and/or sagittal plane, LFT can be modified for greater results. Myofascial Mapping was developed by (Weiselfish) Giammatteo, and is a differential diagnostic technique which localizes areas of neuromusculoskeletal dysfunction, and is taught at courses presented by Dialogues in Contemporary Rehabilitation.

Longitudinal Fiber Therapy for the Guidance System requires the skill *Local Listening*, which was developed by Jean Pierre Barral, D.O., a French osteopathic physician, internationally recognized for his manual therapy approach, Visceral Manipulation. Visceral Manipulation courses are taught in North America under the direction of Frank Lowen. Local Listening is a differential diagnostic technique for finding relationships and patterns of dysfunction.

How to Use the Synchronizer for LFT for the Guidance System

It is difficult to maintain all of the steps above for Longitudinal Fiber Therapy for the Guidance System and at the same time to maintain hand contact on the Synchronizer. The client's hand can be used for contact, or the hand of another (for example, an aide).

SYNCHRONIZER FOR LFT

Three inches caudal to the foramen magnum, from that point, 1 inch lateral.

TREATMENT: PHASE ONE

1. Place a hand over the ligament.
2. Assess: Place longitudinal traction on the ligament in a superior and an inferior direction (i.e., longitudinal stretch). Assess the resistance of: (1) inferior traction, and (2) superior traction.
3. Place longitudinal traction on the ligament in the direction of greater resistance: (1) inferior traction, or (2) superior traction.
4. Then place longitudinal traction (distraction) on the distal bone of ligament attachment close to the articular surface.
5. Then, move the articular surface of the ligament attachment which is now distracted in a longitudinal manner (the distal bone of attachment) in a 3-Planar Fascial Fulcrum approach (developed by (Weiselfish) Giammatteo, presented in Chapter 10 of this text).
6. Maintain the longitudinal traction on the ligament (inferior or superior). Maintain the longitudinal distraction on the distal bone of attachment. Maintain the 3-Planar Articular Fascial Release of the distal bone articular surface.
7. *Maintaining the Fulcrum:* Maintain Step 6 until a complete "Release" is attained.

TREATMENT: PHASE TWO

1. Local Listening from the ligament in dysfunction.
2. Local Listening is performed from the ligament of the dysfunctional joint to other ligaments in the body. Often it is sufficient to scan the extremity, if the ligament in dysfunction is in an extremity joint. If the ligament in dysfunction is in the spine, often it is sufficient to scan the spine. If the thorax and rib cage is the seat of the ligament in dysfunction, it may often be sufficient to scan the total thorax and rib cage.
3. When coronal and/or sagittal plane Myofascial Mapping is positive at the ligament of dysfunction, and when multiple ligaments are involved, it is necessary to scan the total body with Local Listening. When Myofascial Mapping is positive on a transverse plane only at the ligament of dysfunction, it may not be necessary to scan the total body.
4. One hand contacts the ligament in dysfunction. The second hand contacts the ligament/ligaments of positive Local Listening, one ligament at a time.
5. Inhibitory Balance Testing (Chauffour, Mechanical Link) can be performed among the ligaments which are Local Listening positive, in order to discover the primary dominant ligament/ligaments. Inhibitory Balance Testing was developed by Paul Chauffour in order to ascertain which dysfunction of the body overrides other dysfunctions.
6. Perform Neurofascial Process with hand contact on both ligaments. Neurofascial Process was developed by (Weiselfish) Giammatteo for treatment of pain and disability. When this technique is not familiar to the therapist, simply maintain contact with both hands on the two ligaments, until all tissue tension changes during the "Release" subsides.
7. Perform Neurofascial Process among all of the ligaments of the body which are related in a similar pattern, evident with Local Listening.

CHAPTER 15

PRESSURE SENSOR THERAPY

OF THE FOOT AND ANKLE COMPLEX

Integrative Manual Therapy for Pressure Sensor Therapy

The following is a new avenue of therapy appropriate for clients with severe postural deviations of the feet. Included in the recommended program for therapy are the following:

- Strain and Counterstrain to decrease protective muscle spasm and spasticity affecting tone and posture of the foot.
- Myofascial Release to decrease fascial dysfunction of the foot, especially the plantar fascia.
- Muscle Energy and 'Beyond' Technique for the pelvis to improve balance and weight bearing, and for the sacrum to normalize innervation to the foot and ankle, via alleviation of sacral plexus tension.
- Muscle Energy and 'Beyond' Technique for the tibiotalar joint.
- Tendon Release Therapy, especially for the Achilles tendon, peroneal tendons, and tendons of the toes.
- Ligament Fiber Therapy.
- Visceral mobilization to decrease any fascial restrictions of the pelvic and abdominal region which may be affecting the fascial elongation of the leg, foot and ankle.
- Neural Tissue Tension Technique to decrease all fascial restrictions of: the dura mater and dural sheaths; the peripheral nerves including sciatic, tibial, common peroneal; and to address any spinal cord fibrosis.
- Advanced Strain and Counterstrain Technique to address circulation problems of the extremity.

Beyond the fascial, circulatory, bony, articular, muscle, tendinous and ligamentous restrictions which may be affecting the foot and ankle, there are often pressure-related restrictions. When the foot hits the ground, there is a pressure resistance within the foot and ankle complex which forces the foot into a resistance mode. This resistance mode allows the ground forces to "pressurize" (adapt internal pressures) during transcription of forces up the leg. This resistance mode is required for balance. (Weiselfish) Giammatteo discovered Pressure Sensors, and learned that these Pressure Sensors within the foot and ankle complex are often compromised secondary to trauma, tissue damage, and poor postural alignment.

Neurofascial Process

Neurofascial Process (NFP) was developed by (Weiselfish) Giammatteo as a therapeutic process which addresses body/mind process problems. NFP can be adapted for treatment of foot and ankle Pressure Sensors. For example, Step 6, #4: Contact the Pressure Sensor. Contact the other location (e.g., the right greater trochanter). Maintain contact of the two locations until the "Release" is complete. This "Release" may take up to 30 minutes.

Although this protocol, Foot Pressure Therapy, may appear prolonged, it is possible to attain dramatic changes in foot posture, even in the neurologic foot, and to attain significant balance and ambulation function which otherwise might not be forthcoming.

Location of Pressure Sensors of Foot

Location of theses Pressure Sensors within the foot and ankle complex are found specifically at the following places:

Pressure Sensors

- Anterior to the lateral malleolus and 1 mm caudal.
- Posterior to the medial malleolus and 3 mm caudal.
- Five (5) mm distal to each of the three cuneiforms, distal from their distal articular surfaces, exactly midline (medial/lateral midline) of each cuneiform, on the dorsal surface.
- Two (2) mm superior to the proximal articular surface of the first metatarsal head on the dorsal surface.
- Lateral to the proximal head of the fifth metatarsal, on the very lateral surface.

These seven (7) Pressure Sensors resist forces transcribed up the leg during weight bearing. The resultant resistance is the balance of the foot-ground forces.

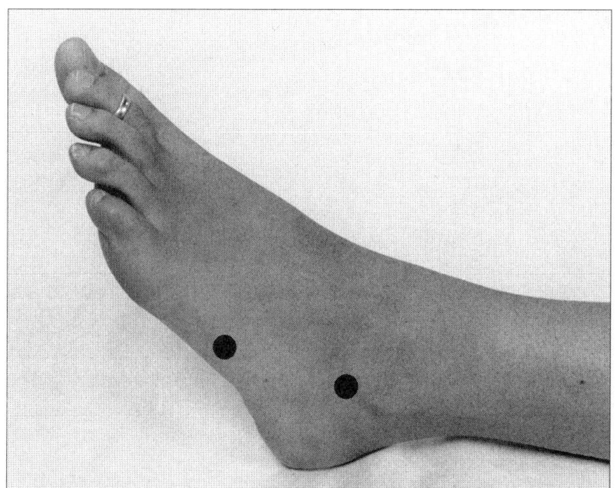

Lateral view of two Pressure Sensors of foot (one is anterior and one (1) mm inferior to lateral malleolus); one is lateral to the proximal head of the fifth metatarsal).

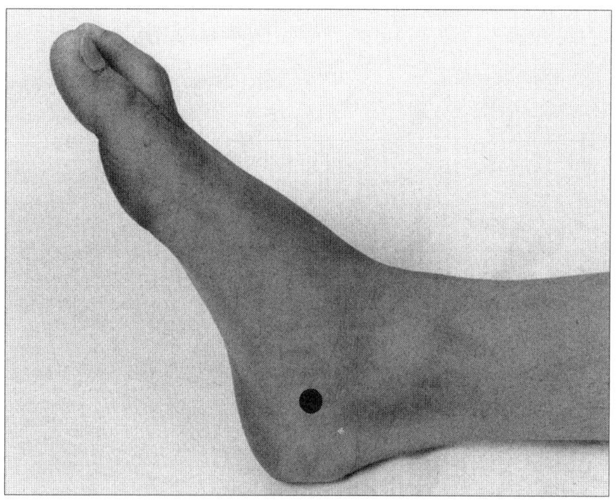

Medial view of one Pressure Sensor of foot (posterior and three (3) mm caudal to medial malleolus).

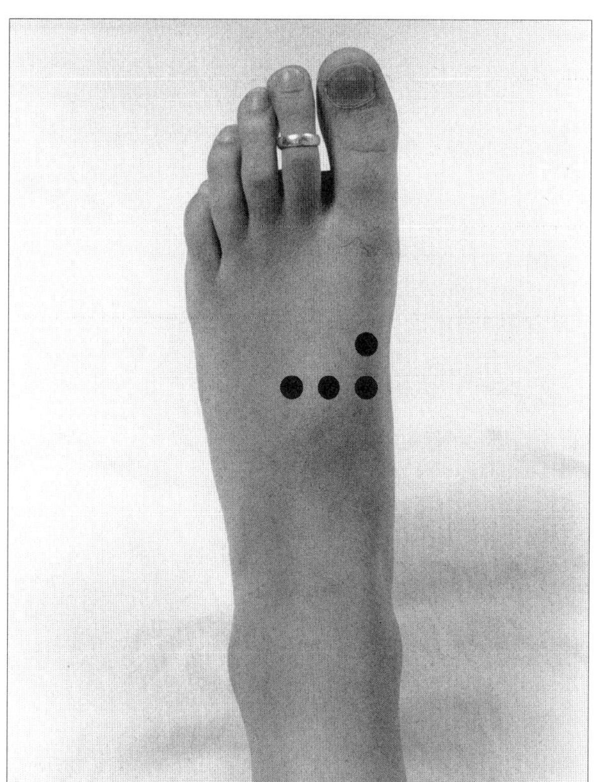

Dorsal view of four Pressure Sensors of foot (three are each five (5) mm distal to each cuneiform, midline; one is two (2) mm superior to proximal first metatarsal head).

Treatment with Foot Pressure Therapy

Treatment of the lower extremity for balance utilizing Pressure Sensors is as follows:

Step 1. Perform a 3-Planar Fascial Fulcrum Soft Tissue Myofascial Release Technique (Chapter 12) with the Pressure Sensors between the two hands to eliminate fascial restrictions surrounding the sensors.

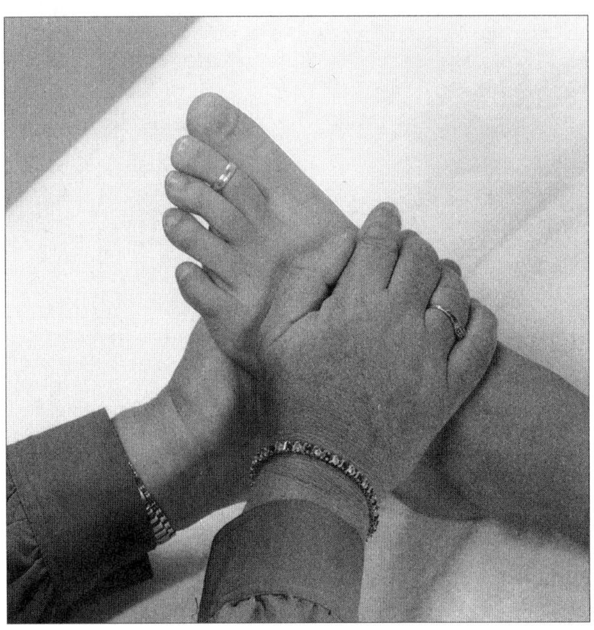

Soft Tissue Myofascial Release Technique, a 3-Planar Fascial Fulcrum Approach, over cuneiform Pressure Sensors.

Step 2. Perform Neurofascial Process (see beginning of chapter): Connect each Pressure Sensor of the foot/ankle complex to the Heart Pressure Sensor which is located at the anterior/inferior heart.

Step 3. Perform Neurofascial Process: Connect each Pressure Sensor to the low back (ureters) to eliminate any toxicity which may be affecting the Pressure Sensors.

Step 4. Perform Neurofascial Process: Connect the Pressure Sensors to:

1. Sacrum
2. T12/L1
3. C7/T1
4. O/A and the transverse sinus

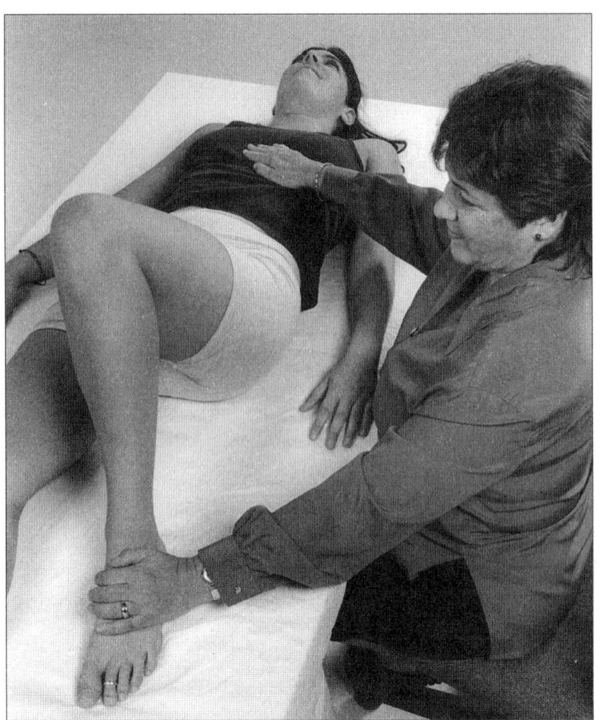

Connect the Pressure Sensors of the foot (cuneiform Pressure Sensors) with the inferior aspect of the heart and wait for the "Release."

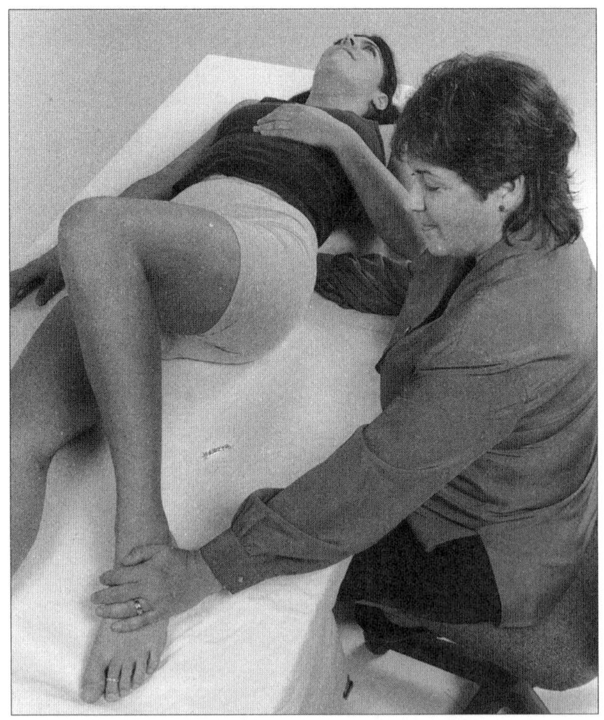

Connect the Pressure Sensors of the foot (cuneiform Pressure Sensors) to the low back and wait for the "Release."

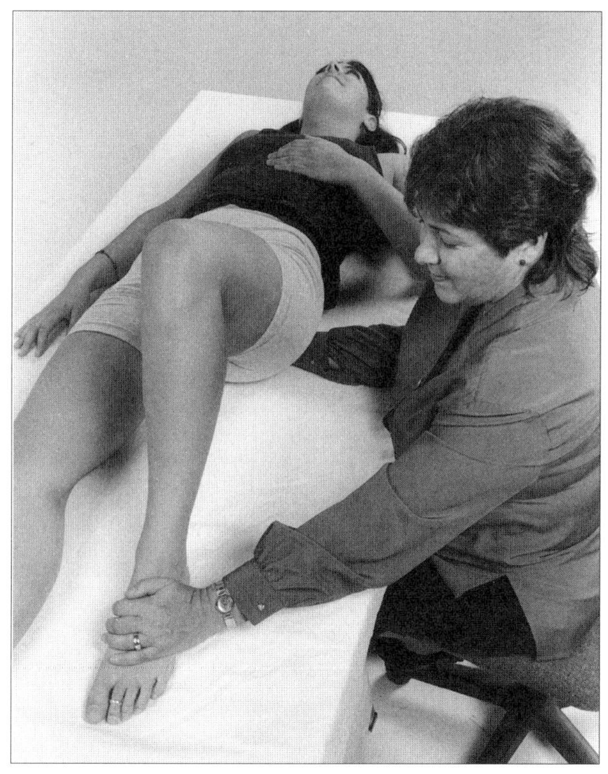

Connect the cuneiform Pressure Sensors with sacrum and wait for the "Release."

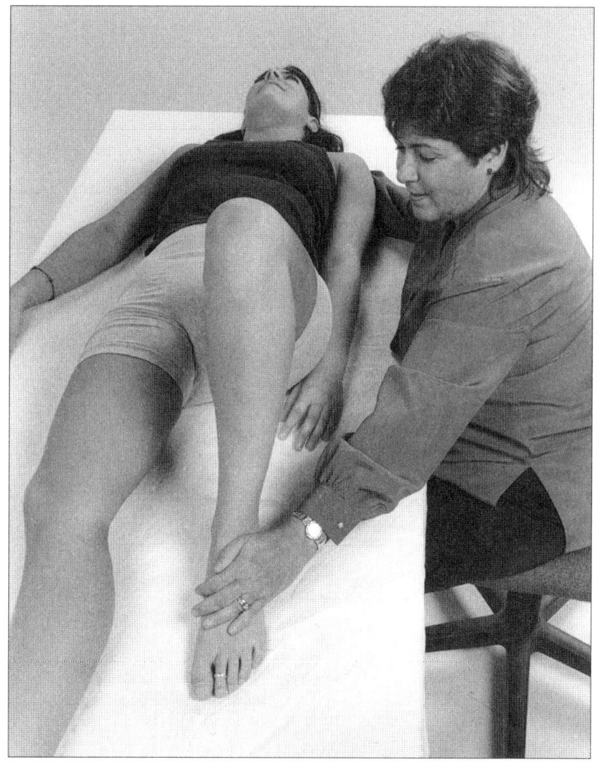

Connect the cuneiform Pressure Sensors with C7/T1 and wait for the "Release."

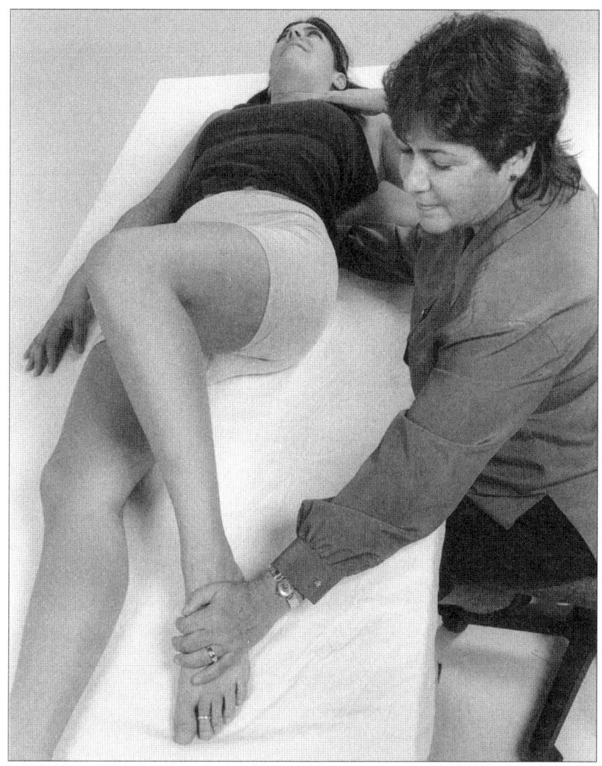

Connect the cuneiform Pressure Sensors with T12/L1 and wait for the "Release."

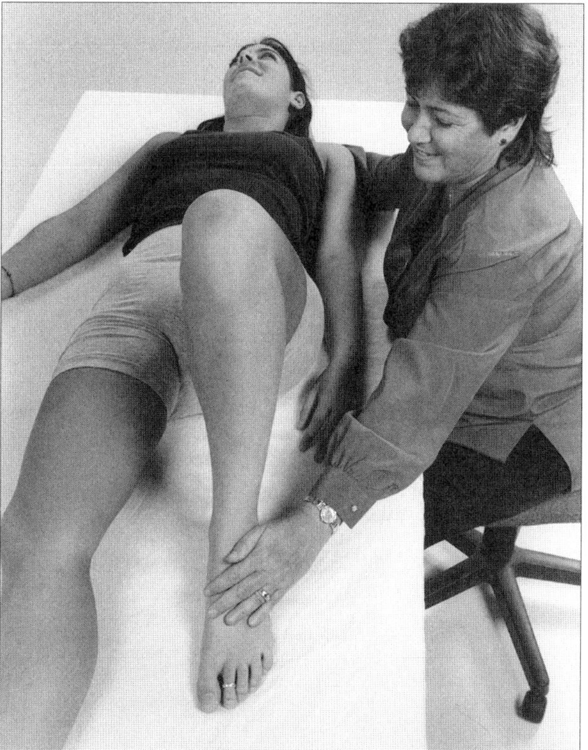

Connect the cuneiform Pressure Sensors with the O/A and transverse sinus and wait for the "Release."

Step 5. Perform Neurofascial Process: Connect each Pressure Sensor to:

1. Pubic/suprapubic region
2. Xiphoid region including lower rib cage and infracostal tissue
3. Anterior thoracic outlet

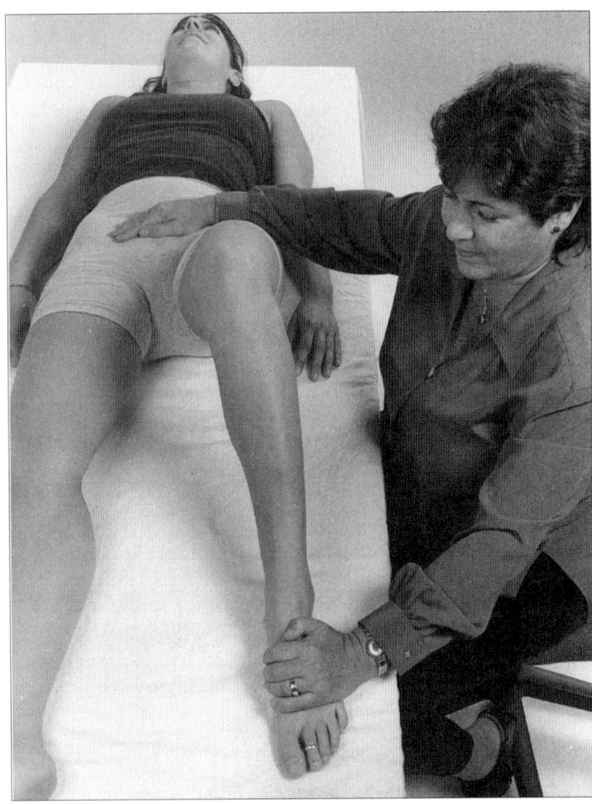

Connect the cuneiform Pressure Sensors with the pubic region and wait for the "Release."

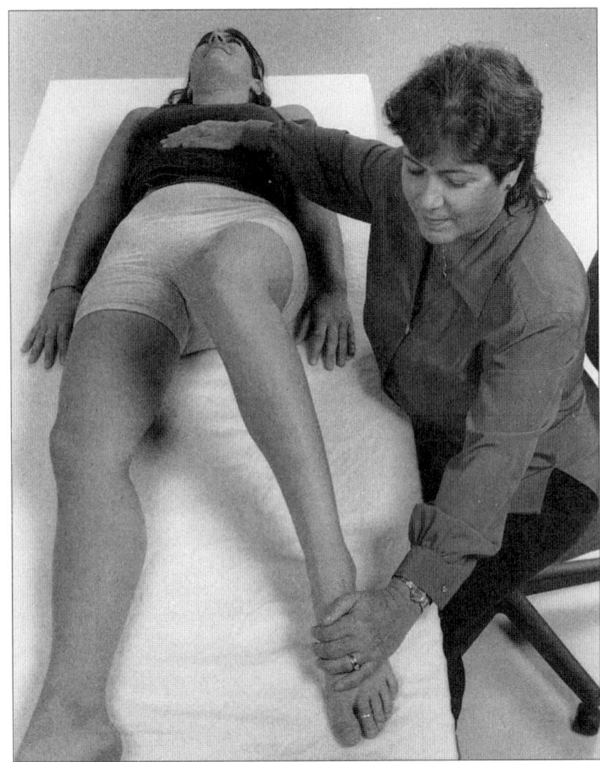

Connect the cuneiform Pressure Sensors with the low sternum and rib cage and wait for the "Release."

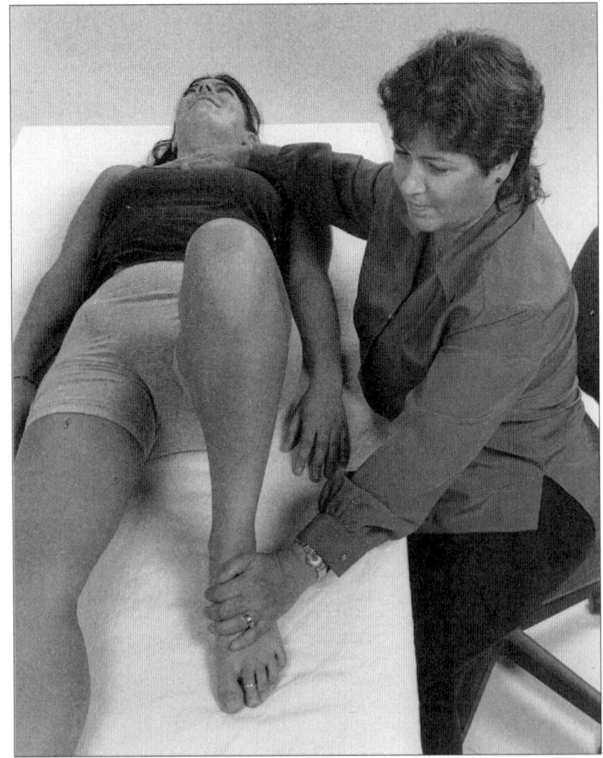

Connect the cuneiform Pressure Sensors with the anterior thoracic outlet and wait for the "Release."

Step 6. Perform Neurofascial Process: Connect each Pressure Sensor:

1. All malleoli
2. Medial tibial plateau
3. Lateral tibial plateau
4. Greater trochanters
5. Ischial tuberosities
6. PSIS bilateral
7. ASIS bilateral
8. Pubic symphysis

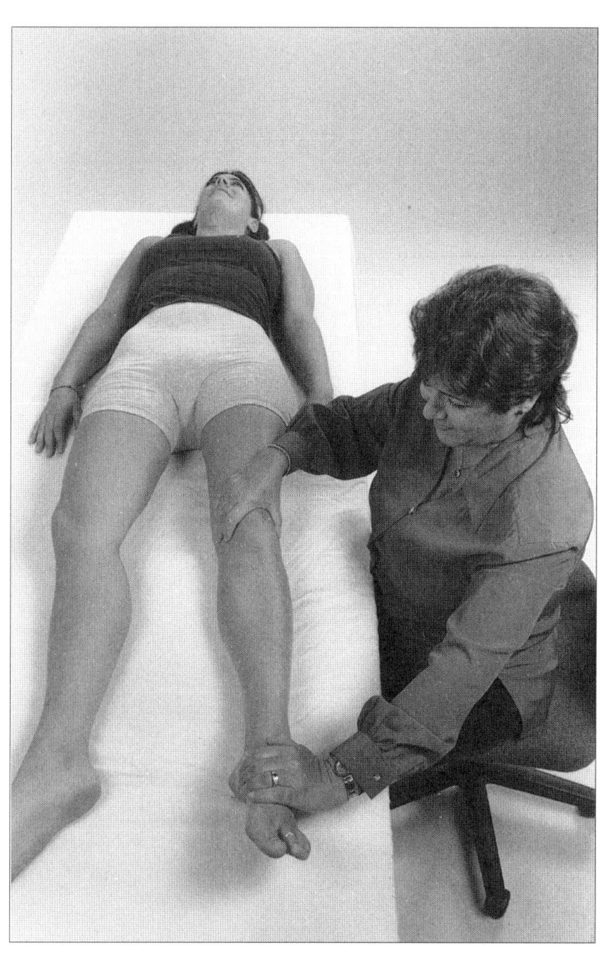

Connect the cuneiform Pressure Sensors to the medial and lateral tibial plateaus and wait for the "Release."

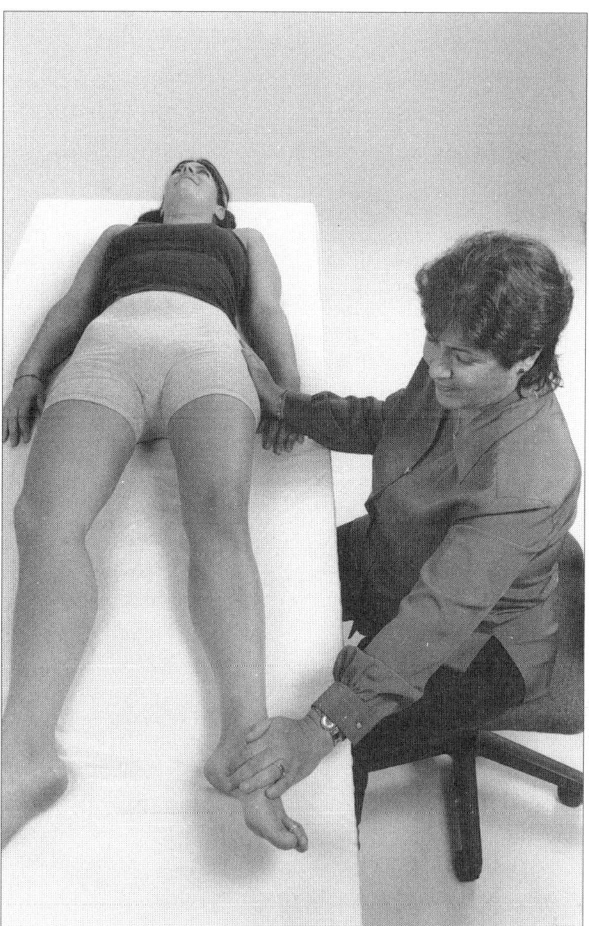

Connect the cuneiform Pressure Sensors to the greater trochanter and wait for the "Release."

CHAPTER 16

REFLEX AMBULATION THERAPY

WITH SYNCHRONIZERS

Gait Requirements for Ambulation

Stance Phase	Heel strike just prior to toe-off of the same extremity.
Initial Contact:	The movement when the extremity meets the ground.
Heel Strike:	Initial contact of the extremity heel with the ground.
Foot Flat:	The foot fully contacts the ground, a loading response secondary to the contralateral extremity beginning swing phase.
Mid-stance:	Body weight passes over the supporting extremity.
Heel-Off:	Heel of the supporting leg leaves the ground just as the contralateral extremity prepares for heel strike.
Toe-Off:	A pre-swing period when only the toe of the supporting extremity is in contact with the ground.
Swing Phase	Toe-off to just prior to heel strike of the same extremity (no contact is made with the ground).
Acceleration:	Begins when the extremity leaves the supporting surface until maximal knee flexion is achieved.
Mid-swing:	The extremity passes directly below the body and the tibia achieves a vertical position.
Deceleration:	The knee is extending in preparation for heel stance and the tibia passes beyond vertical.
Double Support:	Both extremities are in contact with the supporting surface at the same time.
Stride Length:	Distance from the point of heel strike of one extremity to the next heel strike of the same extremity (24 to 169 cm normally in adults).
Stride Duration:	The amount of time to accomplish one stride (0.95 to 1.15 seconds normally in adults).
Step Length:	Distance between two successive points of contact of opposite extremities.
Cadence:	Number of step lengths per minute (90 to 130 steps/minute normally in adults).
Velocity:	Cadence times step length (115 to 171 cm/sec normally in adults).
Base of support:	Distance between one foot and the other (4 to 11.2 cm normally in adults).
Arm swing:	The upper extremities move in a sagittal plane in reciprocation with the lower extremities.
Trunk Counter-rotation:	The trunk rotates in a pattern reciprocally with the lower extremities and contralateral to the upper extremities.

The above information was collated from multiple sources, including research by (Weiselfish) Giammatteo.

This 11-step protocol is time-consuming. Results are worthwhile for the difficult and complex clients. It will facilitate normal ambulation for the first time with cerebral palsy clients, spinal cord clients, and others.

Protocol for Reflex Ambulation Therapy

1. Positive supporting reflex
2. Lumbar regulation
3. Reciprocal mobilities
    - Pelvis and hip joints
    - Pelvis and sacrum
    - Pelvis and L5
    - L5 and sacrum
    - L5 and hips
4. Lumbar thrust
5. Occipitoatlantal traction
6. Occipitosacral traction
7. Leg protective responses
8. Tibiotalar glides
9. Subtalar pressures
10. Flexors: Forces from toes to anterior lumbar flexors.
11. Extensors: Pressures from toe to gluteus and spinal extensors.

Step 1. Positive Supporting Reflex

This reflex is required for all movement when moving downhill, for example, and down steps. When one leg goes first down a step, and the plantar aspect of the metatarsal heads come in contact with the bottom step, the positive supporting reflex is stimulated and the leg can be "stood on." For every intention that ambulation requires, i.e., one foot forward when the other leg is in stance phase, while the swing phase leg is extending towards heel strike and metatarsal strike in descent, there is a positive supporting reflex impression on the extending leg. This means the positive supporting reflex is necessary for going down hills and down steps and down inclines. The positive supporting reflex is also necessary for basic extension of the swing phase leg towards heel strike when walking on a flat surface, up an incline, up steps, and more.

STIMULATION

Supine position:

Stimulation of pressure onto the plantar aspect of the distal metatarsal heads, each head individually and all five metatarsal heads as a unit. This stimulation can continue for ten minutes at a time. The pressure is direct superior pressure onto the metatarsal heads rather than a dorsiflexion pressure which would be torqued.

Sitting position:

Direct superior pressure on the distal metatarsal heads, each head individually and all metatarsal heads together as a unit.

Kneeling position:

Direct superior pressure on the metatarsal heads, each head individually and then all the metatarsal heads together as a unit.

Half-kneeling position:

Direct superior pressure on the metatarsal heads, each head individually and then all the metatarsal heads together as a unit.

Standing position:

Direct superior pressure on the metatarsal heads, each head individually and then all the metatarsal heads together as a unit.

TREATMENT

A half-hour session can consist of this direct pressure on the metatarsal heads, and that will stimulate the positive supporting reflex. In a relatively healthy individual without significant neurologic deficits, one or two treatment sessions of stimulation of the positive supporting reflex should suffice. For patients with significant neurologic deficits, an additional 3 to 5 treatment sessions will be sufficient. It is necessary to progress through the neurodevelopmental milestones with this superior pressure on the metatarsals, and not to miss any of the positions.

Step 2. Lumbar Regulation

Lumbar regulation means the upright position of the spine for standing and ambulation. This requires coordinated and synergistic muscle contraction. It is possible to stimulate this response for clients with significant neurologic deficits.

SYNCHRONIZERS

There is a simple way to perform this process of stimulation of lumbar regulation by using the Synchronizers:

1. *Synchronizer for actin/myosin unlocking/locking mechanisms:* located at the mesosigmoid/sigmoid colon interface.
2. *Synchronizer for tetanic flow of impulses into the motor end plate:* located at either side of the transverse processes of L1, 3 cm lateral to the tips of the transverse processes.

Contact these Synchronizers with the following muscles of the abdominal and lumbar regions to achieve stimulation of lumbar regulation:

1. Abdominals
2. Quadratus lumborum
3. Spinal extensor muscles

Maintain contact on these muscles while at the same time contacting both synchronizers. This may require using the client's hands, as well as the hands of the therapist, and possibly an aide. These can also be contacted one at a time treating each one separately if you don't have enough hands or the client is not able to assist you.

Contact on all muscles of the abdominal and lumbar region is required at the same time as contact is applied to the Synchronizers.

TREATMENT

Periods of 5 minutes up to a half hour are acceptable for this contact. A relatively healthy person will need one treatment session with application of contact for 30 minutes. A client with neurologic deficits may require up to 3 treatment sessions with a half hour of contact applied.

Step 3. Reciprocal Mobilities

Reciprocal mobilities are always 3-planar: sagittal, coronal, and transverse plane together. It is understood ((Weiselfish) Giammatteo) that reciprocal mobility is present at the lumbosacral junction. Research on the Cross Crawl machine has provided evidence of reciprocal mobility on three planes at multiple interfaces of: hard frame to hard frame; hard frame to inner body; inner body to inner body. The reciprocal movements required for ambulation include:

- Pelvis and hip joints
- Pelvic and sacrum joints
- Pelvic and L5
- L5 and sacrum
- L5 and hip joints

This protocol can be used when the client is on the Cross Crawl machine or while the person moves the limbs reciprocally.

SYNCHRONIZER

Synchronizer for stimulating reciprocal motilities: on the medial border of the spine of the left scapula.

Reciprocal Mobilities: When Right Leg is in Stance Phase

Right Hip/Femoral Head

Flexion
Adduction
Internal Rotation

Right Pelvis

Inferior Glide of Ilia Surface
Outflare
External Rotation
Posterior Rotation

Left Hip/Femoral Head

Extension
Abduction
External Rotation

Left Pelvis

Superior Glide of Ilia Surface
Inflare
Internal Rotation
Anterior Rotation

Sacrum

Flexion
Anterior Left Sacral Torsion (LOL)
Left Rotation
Left Side Bending

L5

Extension
Right Rotation
Right Side Bending
Right Facet Closure
Left Facet Opening

TREATMENT

Contact the Synchronizer on the medial border of the spine of the left scapula. The second hand can contact, in sequence: pelvis, L5, hips. These hand contacts occur during ambulation.

Pelvis and Hip Joints

The pelvis and the hips are reciprocal in the following manner: The hip is in flexion as the pelvis is in inferior glide on the same side; the hip is in adduction as the pelvis is in outflare on that same side; the hip is in internal rotation as the pelvis is in external rotation on that same side.

The pelvis does go into a posterior rotation while the hip is flexing. The pelvis goes towards an anterior rotation while the hip is extending, i.e., moves away from posterior rotation. The posterior rotation of the pelvis is a physiologic movement combined with accessory motions of the ilial articular surface which include: inferior glide, outflare, and external rotation. The anterior rotation of the pelvis is the physiologic motion of the ilium which is combined with the accessory movements at the ilial articular surface, which includes: superior glide of the ilial surface, inflare, and internal rotation.

The hip and pelvis are synchronized for reciprocal movement of the femoral head and the ilial articular surface on the ipsilateral side, although there is a co-joining of forces on three planes as there is hip flexion together with posterior rotation of the pelvis and hip extension together with anterior rotation of the pelvis. This means that the physiologic movements of the ilium are in opposite directions of the movements of the joint surface of ilium. This is not unique, an example of which in the upper quadrant is: abduction of the arm while there is inferior glide of the humeral head.

There is reciprocal movement of the right and left sides of the hip/pelvis complex. One hip will flex and adduct and internally rotate, while the opposite hip will extend and abduct and externally rotate.

There is reciprocal movement between the hip and the opposite pelvis in regards to physiologic motion. One hip will flex and adduct and internally rotate, while the opposite pelvis is moving towards anterior rotation. The hip will extend and abduct and externally rotate, while the opposite pelvis is in posterior rotation.

There is a co-joined and synchronous movement between the hip movements of the femoral head, and the movements of the articular surface of ilium on the opposite side. While the femoral head flexes and adducts and internally rotates, the opposite ilial surface will have the following accessory movements: superior glide with inflare and internal rotation.

These hip and pelvic movements are required for stride, and require stimulation, rather than aggressive mobilization and manual therapy. As long as there are free glides at the joints (femoral head with acetabulum), and ilium and pubic symphysis, there is easy stimulation of reciprocal movements of femoral head and pelvis.

Pelvis and Sacrum

The pelvis and sacrum move reciprocally in a physiologic manner. Rather than accessory joint movements being reciprocal, the physiologic motions are reciprocal. This means that anterior and posterior rotation of the pelvis, and flexion and extension of the sacrum are reciprocal. Reciprocal movement occurs at all times and on all three planes. Posterior rotation and anterior rotation of the pelvis are 3-planar motions. Flexion and extension of sacrum are uni-planar motions, but when combined with the lumboscral junction for ambulation, 3-planar motion is evident. Thus, when describing reciprocal movements of the pelvis and sacrum, it is necessary to describe the combined sacroiliac joint flexion and extension together with the lumbosacral junction 3-planar torsions (Reference (Weiselfish) Giammatteo: *Manual Therapy for the Pelvis, Sacrum, Cervical, Thoracic, and Lumbar Spine Emphasizing Muscle Energy Techniques*).

The pelvis will go into posterior rotation as the sacrum flexes and sacral torsion occurs to the opposite side (left sacral torsion means a torsion towards the left side. Right sacral torsion means a torsion to the right side. Left sacral torsion occurs with right posterior rotation. Right sacral torsion occurs with left posterior rotation of the pelvis. The torsion occurs together with the sagittal plane flexion of sacrum.

Ambulation is supposed to occur only with flexion of the sacrum, rather than any sacral extension. Therefore the pelvis should truly be in a posterior rotation, rather than an anterior rotation. The range of posterior rotation is from stance phase (0 degrees) through swing phase, when full posterior rotation of the pelvis occurs. Even during toe-off of stance phase there is a posterior rotation of the pelvis, i.e., the pelvis is not in anterior rotation. The pelvis moves from: 0 percent posterior rotation during toe-off with the leg fully extended, towards 100 percent posterior rotation of the pelvis at mid-swing phase. During swing phase, which occurs when the opposite leg is in mid-stance through toe-off, the pelvis is in 100 percent posterior rotation. The only time a true anterior rotation occurs at the pelvis during stance phase is when biomechanical dysfunction of the pelvis and sacrum is present.

Anterior rotation of the pelvis is really only required during hyperextension of the leg, which does occur during running. During running, there are moments when both feet are off the ground. During extension of the hip, when the foot is on the ground in running, there is anterior rotation of the pelvis.

Pelvis and L5

Sacral flexion occurs together with anterior torsions. The sacrum is always supposed to be flexed during ambulation. During running (as compared to ambulation) there is an abnormal compensation of the body when the pelvis goes into an anterior pelvic rotation, while the hip is hyperextended and the sacrum stays in its flexed position. This is why runners often develop biomechanical dysfunctions of the pelvic joints. Whenever there is a posterior rotation of the pelvis, which includes an inferior glide of the articular surface of ilium together with an outflare and an external rotation of ilium, the facet joints are open on the side of L5 which articulates with the sacral facet. When there is swing phase and the pelvis is moving into full posterior rotation and the articular surface of ilium is gliding inferior with outflare and external rotation at the articular surface, the facet of L5 on that ipsilateral side is opening. As the leg moves from swing phase towards stance phase and continues through stance phase, the pelvis is moving from full posterior rotation towards 0 percent posterior rotation; at the ilial surface, the movement is from an inferior glide towards neutral (in the direction of superior glide) but not going into superior glide, out of outflare (moving towards inflare but not going into inflare), and moving from external rotation going towards internal rotation (but not into internal rotation); the L5 facet is closing on that side. The facet does not have normal 3-planar motion. That is because it is a closing and opening movement. Yet in biomechanics, there is a manifestation of 3-planar movement seen at the facet joint which is cojoined with the vertebral bodies and reciprocal movements of the lumbosacral junction.

L5 and Sacrum

The lumbosacral junction is the junction between L5 and S1. The complexity at this junction is phenomenal. This text will be limited to the reciprocal movements which occur at this junction. As the sacrum flexes, L5 extends. As the sacrum rotates to the right, L5 rotates to the left. As sacrum side bends to the right, L5 side bends to the left. There is no neutral (Type I) movement of the lumbosacral junction. L5 relative to S1 is always in "lumbosacral extension," which means L5 is extended and sacral base is flexed (anterior glide of sacral base). This is evolution for purposes of protection of the L5 disc, which maintains the hydrostatic pressure for anterior presence of the disc whenever L5 is extended. There is only Type II movement at the lumbosacral junction which means when sacrum is flexed and L5 is extended; this is lumbosacral extension. When sacrum is extended and L5 is flexed, this is lumbosacral flexion.

During ambulation, lumbosacral extension is maintained. This protects the disc at all times. During stance phase when forces are transcribed up the leg, there is an anterior torsion to the opposite side. When the right leg is in stance phase, there is a left sacral torsion. When there is a left sacral torsion, sacrum is flexed and rotated to the left and side bent to the left. When there is a left sacral torsion, during right stance phase, L5 is extended and rotated to the right and side bent to the right. There is closure of the right facet. The hydrostatic pressure within the disc will cause pressure of the disc material on the left side. The right stance phase forces which are transcribed from the ground up the leg will not place undue pressures on the disc, which are now at the left side of the intervertebral body space.

During running, there is occasionally an extension of sacrum and a flexion of L5. Therefore running can cause discogenic problems to occur. During ambulation, this is not the case.

L5 and Hips

L5 and the hips move in reciprocal mobility during ambulation. When the femoral head flexes and internally rotates and adducts, there is an opening of the facet on the contralateral side. When the femoral head extends and abducts and externally rotates, there is a closing of the facet on the contralateral side.

Step 4. Lumbar Thrust

Lumbar thrust is momentum focused from the lumbosacral junction and determined according to velocity as well as amplitude of forward stride. The lumbar thrust is the momentum which carries the spine forward during ambulation.

The lumbar thrust utilizes these essential muscles:

- Iliacus
- Psoas major
- Psoas minor
- Quadratus lumborum
- Latissimus dorsi
- Abdominals—including external and internal obliques

SYNCHRONIZERS

Maintain the isometric resistance with contact on the Synchronizers:

1. *Synchronizer for actin/myosin unlocking/locking mechanisms:* located at the mesosigmoid/sigmoid colon interface.
2. *Synchronizer for tetanic flow of impulses into the motor end plate:* located at either side of the transverse processes of L1, 3cm lateral to the tips of the transverse processes.

TREATMENT

The lumbar thrust can be treated for depleted strength and force in the following manner:

1. Treat the client in the supine position, in the sitting position, and then in the standing position.
2. Perform isometric resistance to the lumbar thrust motion
3. Maintain the isometric resistance with the contact on the Synchronizer for 10 repetitions of 10 seconds.
4. This can be performed daily.

A healthy client without neurologic deficits is able to stimulate lumbar thrust within 1 week if this protocol is performed 10 repetitions daily for 10 second isometric resistances, with contact on the Synchronizers. The client with neurologic deficits may need 10 to 20 sessions, not more than 1 week apart.

Step 5. Occipitoatlantal Traction

Occipitoatlantal traction is the maintenance of the head on the neck, aligned in a perpendicular fashion to the base of support and the vectors through the eyes and ears and mastoid processes parallel to the floor.

In order to facilitate what could be called "head control" during ambulation, there is a Synchronizer at the parietals which will stimulate occipitoatlantal traction.

SYNCHRONIZER

Synchronizer for Head Control: located on both parietals, 3 inches posterior from the coronal suture and one inch lateral from the sagittal suture.

TREATMENT

The Synchronizer can be held during sitting with head control maintained (passive, progressing to assisted active, progressing to active, progressing to resisted). Progress to standing and ambulation.

The patient can be treated in the sitting and in the standing and in the walking modes for facilitation of the occipitoatlantal traction during ambulation, with contact on the Synchronizer while these positions are maintained. Treatment sessions can be up to 10 minutes. A healthy person without neurologic deficits requires 2 or 3 treatment sessions for healthy head control during ambulation. A patient with neurologic deficits may need 5 to 10 treatment sessions of 10 to 20 minutes.

Step 6. Occipitosacral Traction

Occipitosacral traction is the maintenance of distance between occiput and sacral base during standing and ambulation.

SYNCHRONIZERS

Synchronizers for Stimulation of Occipitosacral Traction:

1. Located on the parietals 1 3/4 inches posterior from the coronal suture.
2. Located 3/4 of an inch lateral from the sagittal suture on both sides.

TREATMENT

Occipitosacral traction can be stimulated during sitting, standing and then ambulation. The distance between occiput and sacrum can be maintained with body traction with contact maintained on both Synchronizers while ambulating in the following order:

1. Passive
2. Active-assisted
3. Active
4. Resisted

A healthy person may require 10 minute sessions, 3 to 5 repetitions. A person with neurologic deficits may require 10 minute sessions for 5 to 10 repetitions.

Step 7. Leg Protective Responses

Leg protective responses are the maintained supporting mechanisms of a pull-like nature, which allow us to stand on one foot or both feet in stance phase, without collapse at the hips and/or knees and/or ankles. These are reflexes not well documented in literature. They are necessary for standing and ambulation.

SYNCHRONIZER

Synchronizer for Stimulation of Leg Protective Responses: located on the parietal lobes, 1 inch posterior to the coronal sutures and 1 to 1/2 inches lateral from the sagittal suture.

TREATMENT

To stimulate leg protective responses, the person can be treated with contact on the Synchronizers in this order:

1. In the supine position;
2. In the sitting position (with an extended leg and extended hip, i.e., anatomic neutral);
3. In the standing position.

The hip and ankle should be maintained in anatomic neutral with contact on both Synchronizers for 10 minute periods. Treatment can progress in this order:

1. Passive anatomic neutral of leg;
2. Assisted active with maintained anatomic neutral of the leg;
3. Active anatomic neutral of the leg;
4. Resisted maintenance of anatomic neutral of the leg.

A healthy person will require 4 to 5 repetitions of 10 minute treatment sessions. A patient with neurologic deficits may require 5 to 20 repetitions of 10 minute treatment sessions, depending on the nature, chronicity, and severity of the neurologic deficits.

Step 8. Tibiotalar Glides

The tibia glides anterior over talus from mid stance through initiation of push-off until the toe begins to take pressure from the ground.

There is a requirement of 10 degrees dorsiflexion for tibiotalar glides to occur. It is common for fixations (joint dysfunction with protective muscle spasm and fascial dysfunction) to be present with decrease in dorsiflexion, in the majority of the population of healthy and ill persons.

When dorsiflexion is restored (i.e., there is passive dorsiflexion of 10 degrees) then tibiotalar glides may be stimulated.

There are Synchronizers for stimulation of tibiotalar glides which are located at the pelvis.

SYNCHRONIZER

Synchronizers for stimulation of Tibiotalar Glide: located on the tip of the ASIS.

TREATMENT

Tibiotalar glides can be stimulated with contact on the Synchronizers. The tibia can be positioned anterior on talus in the following progression of these positions with contact on the Synchronizers:

1. Supine position
2. Sitting position
3. Standing position
4. Ambulation

The tibia can be maintained anterior to talus in this order:

1. Passively
2. Assisted actively
3. Resisted

Treatment sessions can be 10 minutes duration. The healthy person requires 2 to 3 repetitions of 10 minutes duration. A client with neurologic deficits may require 5 to 20 repetitions of 10 minute treatment sessions.

Step 9. Subtalar Pressures

Subtalar pressures are the cushion effect between talus and calcaneus that allow movement between the ground and the foot, and the heel and leg.

The talocalcaneal joint (subtalar joint) has the momentum/push-off effect for decompression of joints during stance phase.

In order to stimulate the subtalar cushion effect, Synchronizers can be used.

SYNCHRONIZER

Synchronizers for stimulation of subtalar pressures: located on both sides of the pelvis, 1 inch anterior to the greater trochanter and 1/2 inch superior from that point.

TREATMENT

Traction can be maintained on calcaneus for distraction of the talocalcaneal joint, while the Synchronizers are contacted. This distraction and Synchronizer contact can be maintained for 10 minutes duration per treatment session. This can be performed in the following order of progression:

1. Supine
2. Sitting
3. Standing
4. Ambulation

During standing and sitting, a superior traction from talus can be maintained with contact on the Synchronizers. During ambulation, the joint is not distracted; only the Synchronizers are contacted. For the healthy person, 3 to 5 repetitions of 10 minute treatment sessions are required. A client with neurologic deficits may require 5 to 25 repetitions of 10 minute treatment sessions depending on the nature, chronicity, and severity of the neurologic deficits.

Step 10. Flexors

The flexors are used for mid-stance to swing phase, as control/force projectors of movement.

The flexors include the toe flexors, plantar flexors, knee flexors, hip flexors, and anterior lumbar flexors.

The focused and synergistic flexor effect can be stimulated with Synchronizers, which are located on the pelvis.

SYNCHRONIZERS

Synchronizers for stimulation of flexors: located 1 inch lateral from the pubic symphysis and 3 inches superior from that point.

TREATMENT

The following flexor muscle groups can be contacted with the Synchronizer:

1. Lumbar flexors
2. Hip flexors
3. Knee flexors
4. Plantar flexors
5. Toe flexors

It is better to have enough hands available so that all muscle bellies can be contacted at the same time as there is Synchronizer contact. Treatment should progress in the following order of positions:

1. Supine with hip, knee, and ankle flexed
2. Sitting
3. Standing with some leg and lumbar flexion

Treatment sessions are 10 minutes in duration. For the healthy person, 5 to 10 repetitions of 10 minute treatment sessions are required. A client with significant neurologic deficits may require 10 to 25 repetitions of 10 minute treatment sessions.

Step 11. Extensors

The extensors are the pressure/control forces from mid swing-phase to mid-stance. They are the forces of stability rather than mobility.

The extensors place pressure from the toes to the gluteus and spinal extensors.

There are Synchronizers which can stimulate the pressure/force effect during ambulation.

SYNCHRONIZER

Synchronizer for stimulation of extensors: located 1 inch inferior from the PSIS and 3 inches lateral from that point on both sides.

TREATMENT

To stimulate this pressure/force phenomenon, the extensors that can be contacted include:

1. Toe extensors
2. Dorsiflexors
3. Knee extensors
4. Hip extensors
5. Lumbar extensors

During contact on the extensors, the Synchronizers are contacted for stimulation of this stability mode. It is best to have enough hands available during treatment so that all extensor surfaces can be contacted while the Synchronizers are contacted. The treatment can progress in this order of positions:

1. Supine with extended leg and dorsiflexion
2. Sitting with straight leg and dorsiflexion and extended hip
3. Standing
4. Ambulation

During these positions, the Synchronizers are contacted as well as the extensor surfaces of the leg.

CHAPTER 17

PROCEDURES AND PROTOCOLS

TO CORRECT UPPER AND LOWER EXTREMITY DYSFUNCTION WITH INTEGRATIVE MANUAL THERAPY

This chapter lists procedures and protocols for a variety of different dysfunctions in the body. These protocols are recommendations for how to treat these dysfunctions with Integrative Manual Therapy. Much of the treatment techniques listed in this chapter are referenced and taught in this textbook. Some of the techniques listed here are not taught in this text. Further learning on these techniques can be attained through educational materials from Dialogues in Contemporary Rehabilitation, including: Myofascial Release ((Weiselfish) Giammatteo) and Muscle Energy and 'Beyond' Technique ((Weiselfish) Giammatteo). These treatment techniques can be found in textbooks and videos as well as seminars taught by DCR.

Peripheral Joint Dysfunction

ASSESSMENT

Evaluation of the client's objective findings is required prior to therapy. Assessment may include:

- Posture: sagittal plane, coronal plane, transverse plane of the spine.
- Posture: sagittal plane, coronal plane, transverse plane of the extremities.
- Neurologic testing, including dermatome, myotome, and scleratome which is appropriate for the pain and/or disability manifested by the client.
- Functional capacity testing for functional impairments.
- Joint mobility testing of all appropriate joints.
- Ranges of motion of spine and extremity joints.
- Myofascial Mapping ((Weiselfish) Giammatteo).
- Local Listening (Barral).
- Inhibitory Balance Testing (Chauffour).

Therapy for peripheral joints of the arms and legs is almost always appropriate after spine has been assessed. Treat the pelvis, sacrum, spine and rib cage first. The biomechanical function of the peripheral joints is dependent on the biomechanical function of the pelvis, sacrum and spine. It is highly recommended that pelvis and sacrum joints are treated for biomechanical dysfunction before other joints are treated, unless treatment is inhibited for some reason. Muscle Energy and 'Beyond' Technique for the pelvis, sacrum and spine is suggested as exceptional intervention to attain structural integrity of pelvis, sacrum and spine.

TREATMENT

1. Muscle Energy and 'Beyond' Technique for the dysfunctional joint(s). It is often preferable to treat the whole extremity/extremities when there is decreased vertical dimension of only one of the intra-articular spaces. (Chapter 3 and Chapter 4)
2. Eliminate protective muscle spasm with Strain and Counterstrain: Lower quadrant and/or upper quadrant with Synergic Pattern Release. (Chapter 10 and Chapter 11)
3. Myofascial Release:
   - Soft Tissue Myofascial Release: Treat the total extremity where the joint dysfunction is present. (Chapter 12)
   - Articular Fascial Release of the dysfunctional joint/joints. (Chapter 12)
   - Specialized Fascial Release Techniques (Myofascial Release, (Weiselfish) Giammatteo with Dialogues in Contemporary Rehabilitation), for example: scar releases, muscle belly releases. (Not presented in book.)
4. Tendon Release Therapy of the tendons surrounding the joint. (Chapter 13)
5. Ligament Fiber Therapy:
   - Horizontal Fiber Therapy (Chapter 12)
   - Longitudinal Fiber Therapy: Phase One and Phase Two. (Chapter 12)

Total Hip Replacement

ASSESSMENT

- Neurologic and gait
- Ranges of physiologic motion: lumbosacral region, hip, knee, ankle
- Mobility testing of accessory movements: knee joint
- Manual muscle testing
- Protective muscle spasm (muscle barriers): lumbar flexors, iliacus, adductors, abductors, medial hamstrings, quadriceps, gastrocnemius
- Myofascial testing: pelvic diaphragm, hip, thigh, knee: Myofascial Mapping, fascial glide
- Foot posture

TREATMENT

Acute Stage (before 10 days post-op):

1. Myofascial Release:
   - Soft Tissue Myofascial Release: transverse diaphragms (all)
   - Soft Tissue Myofascial Release: knee
2. Muscle Energy and 'Beyond' Technique: bilateral lower extremity joints

Chronic Stage (any time after 10 days post-op):

1. Myofascial Release:
   - Soft Tissue Myofascial Release: transverse diaphragms
   - Soft Tissue Myofascial Release: hip
   - Soft Tissue Myofascial Release: knee
2. Muscle Energy Technique and 'Beyond' for bilateral lower extremity joints
3. Eliminate protective muscle spasm with Strain and Counterstrain:
   - Iliacus
   - Medial hamstrings
   - Anterior fifth lumbar
   - Abductors
   - Adductors (without overpressure)
   - Gastrocnemius
   - Quadriceps
4. Repeat #3
5. Articular Fascial Release: pelvic joints
6. Articular Fascial Release: knee joint
7. Tendon Release Therapy: bilateral lower extremity joints (hold for De-Facilitated Fascial Release)
8. Restore ankle dorsiflexion: mobilize subtalar and tibiotalar joints (Do not place forces on hip.)
9. Ligament Fiber Therapy: bilateral lower extremity joints
10. Orthotics and strengthening

Total Knee Replacement

ASSESSMENT

- Neurologic and gait
- Ranges of physiologic motion: lumbosacral region, hip, knee, ankle
- Mobility testing of accessory movements: hip joint
- Manual muscle testing
- Protective muscle spasm (muscle barriers): lumbar flexors, iliacus, adductors, abductors, medial hamstrings, quadriceps, gastrocnemius
- Myofascial testing: pelvic diaphragm, hip, thigh, knee, ankle: Myofascial Mapping, fascial glide
- Foot posture

TREATMENT

Acute Stage (before 10 days post-op):

1. Myofascial Release:
    - Soft Tissue Myofascial Release: transverse diaphragms (all)
    - Soft Tissue Myofascial Release: hip
    - Soft Tissue Myofascial Release: ankle
2. Muscle Energy and 'Beyond' Technique: bilateral lower extremity joints

Chronic Stage (any time after 10 days post-op):

1. Myofascial Release:
    - Soft Tissue Myofascial Release: transverse diaphragms
    - Soft Tissue Myofascial Release: hip
    - Soft Tissue Myofascial Release: knee
    - Soft Tissue Myofascial Release: ankle
2. Muscle Energy and 'Beyond' Technique: bilateral lower extremity joints
3. Eliminate protective muscle spasm with Strain and Counterstrain:
    - Iliacus
    - Medial hamstrings
    - Anterior fifth lumbar
    - Abductors
    - Adductors
    - Quadriceps
    - Gastrocnemius
4. Repeat #3
5. Articular Fascial Release: pelvic joints
6. Articular Fascial Release: hip joint
7. Tendon Release Therapy: bilateral lower extremity joints (hold for De-Facilitated Fascial Release)
8. Restore ankle dorsiflexion: mobilize subtalar and tibiotalar joints (Do not place forces on knee.)
9. Ligament Fiber Therapy: bilateral lower extremity joints
10. Orthotics and strengthening

Chondromalacia

ASSESSMENT

- Neurologic and gait
- Ranges of physiologic motions: knee
- Mobility testing of accessory movements: knee
- Ligamentous integrity
- Meniscus testing
- Patella Mobility testing
- Apprehension/grinding test for chondromalacia (crepitus: mild, moderate, severe)
- Manual muscle testing
- Leg muscle length: hamstrings, quadriceps, gastrocnemious, adductors, iliotibial band
- Protective muscle spasm (muscle barriers): hip, knee, ankle
- Myofascial test: shins
- Range of physiologic motion: ankle
- Myofascial testing: Myofascial Mapping, fascial glide
- Mobility testing: tibiotalar, subtalar, tibiofibular
- Foot posture: pronation, supination
- Intrinsic foot muscle spasm
- Foot posture

TREATMENT

1. Normalize ankle range of motion: manipulate tibiotalar and subtalar joints.
2. Muscle Energy and 'Beyond' Technique: bilateral lower extremity joints
3. Eliminate protective muscle spasm with Strain and Counterstrain:
   - especially iliacus
   - Hamstrings
   - Anterior and posterior cruciates
   - Quadriceps
   - Medial gastrocnemius
4. Myofascial Release:
   - Soft Tissue Myofascial Release: knee
   - Articular Fascial Release: knee
   - Articular Fascial Release: patellar technique
   - Muscle Belly Technique: quadriceps
   - Muscle Belly Technique: gastrocnemius
5. Patellofemoral mobilization (if residual crepitus is significant):
   - Home rental electrical muscle stimulator with electrode on the distal head of the quadriceps medialis.
   - Use two times a day for 30 minute sessions.
   - Rental for 6 weeks (mild) to 3 months (severe crepitus).
6. Tendon Release Therapy: bilateral lower extremity joints (hold for De-Facilitated Fascial Release)
7. Ligament Fiber Therapy: bilateral lower extremity joints
8. Orthotics:
   - Immediate fabrication of temporary orthotics to normalize forces transcribed up the leg due to pronated or supinated feet.
   - Fabrication of permanent orthotics after completion of Integrative Manual Therapy protocol.
9. Strengthening Program:
   - After elimination of all pain (4 to 6 weeks), give home exercise program to strengthen all pelvic/hip/lower extremity musculature.
   - Quadriceps should wait until completion of Integrative Manual Therapy protocol.

COMMENTS

Four to 10 sessions may be needed to normalize range of motion, eliminate muscle spasm, eliminate pain and inflammation, and treat myofascial dysfunction. Patient may then be checked every 3 to 4 weeks.

Meniscus Dysfunction

ASSESSMENT

- Neurologic and gait
- Ranges of physiologic motions: hip, knee and ankle
- Mobility testing of accessory movements: hip, knee, patella, ankle, tibiofibular
- Compression and locking tests for meniscus; drawer tests
- Manual muscle testing
- Leg muscle length: hamstrings, quadriceps, gastrocnemius, adductors, iliotibial band
- Protective muscle spasm (muscle barriers): iliacus, quadriceps, adductors, abductors, medial hamstrings, gastrocnemius
- Myofascial testing: around knee joint: Myofascial Mapping, fascial glide
- Foot posture: pronation, supination

TREATMENT

1. Muscle Energy and 'Beyond' Technique: bilateral lower extremity joints
2. Eliminate protective muscle spasm with Strain and Counterstrain:
    - Iliacus
    - Adductors
    - Quadriceps
    - Gastrocnemius
3. Myofascial Release:
    - Soft Tissue Myofascial Release: knee joint
    - Articular Fascial Release: tibiofemoral joint
4. Normalize ankle range of motion: manipulate tibiotalar and subtalar joints
5. Eliminate foot and ankle protective muscle spasm with Strain and Counterstrain:
    - Medial ankle
    - Medial calcaneus (foot intrinsics)
6. Myofascial Release—specific Fascial Release Techniques:
    - Medial and lateral collateral ligaments
    - Patella release
    - Muscle Belly Technique: medial hamstrings
    - Muscle Belly Technique: quadriceps
    - Muscle Belly Technique: gastrocnemius
7. Tendon Release Therapy: bilateral lower extremity joints (hold for De-Facilitated Fascial Release)
8. Ligament Fiber Therapy: bilateral lower extremity joints
9. Orthotics and strengthening

Shin Splints

ASSESSMENT

- Neurologic and gait
- Ranges of physiologic motions: knee and ankle
- Mobility testing of accessory movements: knee, ankle, and tibiofibular joints
- Manual muscle testing
- Protective muscle spasm (muscle barriers). Focus: gastrocnemius and tibialis anterior
- Myofascial test: shins: Myofascial Mapping, fascial glide
- Intrinsic foot muscle spasm

TREATMENT

1. Normalize ankle range of motion: manipulate tibiotalar and subtalar joints
2. Eliminate protective muscle spasm with Strain and Counterstrain:
   - Iliacus
   - Hamstrings
   - Abductors
   - Iliotibial band
   - Medial gastrocnemius
   - Lateral ankle
   - Lateral calcaneus
3. Myofascial Release:
   - Soft Tissue Myofascial Release: knee joint
   - Soft Tissue Myofascial Release: anterior compartment (shins)
   - Hanging Technique: tibiofibular joint
   - Muscle Belly Technique: tibialis peroneals
4. Muscle Energy and 'Beyond' Technique: bilateral lower extremity joints
5. Tendon Release Therapy: bilateral lower extremity joints (hold for De-Facilitated Fascial Release)
6. Ligament Fiber Therapy for bilateral lower extremity joints
7. Electrotherapy: Iontophoresis with Iodex (iodine methyl salicylate) to anterior compartment (1 to 4 sessions)
8. Orthotics: assess feet for pronation/supination
9. Strengthening program

COMMENT

2 to 4 sessions is sufficient for shin splints protocol.

Achilles Tendon Tears

ASSESSMENT

- Neurologic and gait
- Ranges of physiologic motions: knee and ankle
- Mobility testing of accessory movements: knee, ankle, and tibiofibular joints
- Manual muscle testing
- Protective muscle spasm (muscle barriers): iliacus, adductors, medial hamstrings, quadriceps, gastrocnemius
- Myofascial testing: around ankle joint, Achilles tendon, calcaneal insertion, gastrocnemius, knee joint (especially posterior aspect): Myofascial Mapping, fascial glide
- Foot posture

TREATMENT

1. Muscle Energy and 'Beyond' Technique: bilateral lower extremity joints
2. Eliminate protective muscle spasm with Strain and Counterstrain:
    - Iliacus
    - Adductors
    - Medial hamstrings
    - Gastrocnemius
3. Myofascial Release:
    - Soft Tissue Myofascial Release: just above site
    - Scar Release: site of tendon tear (after healing)
    - Tendon Release: insertion of tendon on calcaneus
    - Muscle Belly Technique: gastrocnemius
4. Tendon Release Therapy: bilateral lower extremity joints (hold for De-Facilitated Fascial Release)
5. Normalize ankle range of motion: manipulate tibiotalar and subtalar joints
6. Ligament Fiber Therapy for bilateral lower extremity joints
7. Orthotics and strengthening
8. Electrotherapy: iontophoresis with Iodex (iodine methyl salicylate) to anterior compartment (1 to 4 sessions)
9. Orthotics: assess feet for pronation/supination
10. Strengthening program

COMMENT

2 to 4 sessions is sufficient for the Achilles tendon tear protocol.

Plantar Fasciitis

ASSESSMENT

- Neurologic and gait
- Ranges of physiologic motions: ankle and foot
- Mobility testing of accessory movements: ankle and foot joints
- Manual muscle testing
- Protective muscle spasm (muscle barriers): focus on: gastrocnemius, intrinsic foot muscles
- Myofascial testing: plantar fascia: Myofascial Mapping, fascial glide
- Foot posture: pronation, supination

TREATMENT

1. Mobilize ankle range of motion: manipulate tibiotalar and subtalar joints
2. Muscle Energy and 'Beyond' Technique: bilateral lower extremity joints
3. Eliminate protective muscle spasm with Strain and Counterstrain:
    - Iliacus
    - Medial hamstrings
    - Gastrocnemius
    - Flexed calcaneus
    - Intrinsic foot muscles—especially extensors
4. Soft Tissue Myofascial Release: plantar fascia
5. Tendon Release Therapy: bilateral lower extremity joints (hold for De-Facilitated Fascial Release)
6. Ligament Fiber Therapy: bilateral lower extremity joints
7. Orthotics and strengthening program for intrinsics

Spasticity of Lower Quadrant

ASSESSMENT

- Neurologic: focus on spastic synergic pattern which includes:
    - Elevated and retracted pelvis
    - Flexed lumbar and hip
    - Internally rotated hip
    - Flexed (occasionally extended) hip
    - Equinus (plantar flexed) or equinovarus (plantar flexed and inverted) foot
- Gait
- Ranges of physiologic motions: lumbosacral region: hip, knee, ankle
- Mobility testing of accessory joint movements: L5/S1, pelvic joints, hip joint, knee joint, ankle joint
- Muscle tone and muscle testing
- Hypertonicity: lumbar flexors, iliacus, adductors, abductors, medial hamstrings, quadriceps, gastrocnemius
- Myofascial testing: total lower quadrant: Myofascial Mapping, fascial glide
- Foot posture

TREATMENT

1. Eliminate protective muscle spasm with Strain and Counterstrain:
    - All 7 sacral Tender Points
    - Piriformis
    - Anterior fifth lumbar
    - Iliacus
    - Adductors
    - Medial hamstrings
    - Quadriceps
    - Abductors
    - Gastrocnemius
    - Medial ankle
    - Medial calcaneus
    - Lateral ankle
    - Lateral calcaneus (talus for club foot and pronated foot)
2. Myofascial Release:
    - Soft Tissue Myofascial Release: transverse diaphragms (all)
    - Soft Tissue Myofascial Release: hip
    - Soft Tissue Myofascial Release: ankle
    - Soft Tissue Myofascial Release: foot
    - Articular Fascial Release: pelvic joints
    - Articular Fascial Release: hip
    - Articular Fascial Release: knee (tibiofemoral)
    - Articular Fascial Release: ankle (tibiotalar)
    - Muscle Belly Technique: medial hamstrings
    - Muscle Belly Technique: quadriceps
    - Muscle Belly Technique: gastrocnemius
3. Muscle Energy and 'Beyond' Technique: bilateral lower extremity joints
4. Tendon Release Therapy: bilateral lower extremity joints (hold for De-Facilitated Fascial Release)
5. Normalize ankle joint range of motion: manipulate tibiotalar and subtalar joints
6. Ligament Fiber Therapy: bilateral lower extremity joints
7. Repeat #1 and #2
8. Orthotics

Cervical Syndrome

ASSESSMENT

- Posture: sagittal, coronal, transverse planes: total body, focus upper quadrant
- Neurologic: focus upper quadrant
- Ranges of physiologic motions: all upper quadrant joints
- Mobility testing of accessory movements: all upper quadrant joints
- Ligamentous integrity
- Apprehension/grinding tests
- Manual muscle testing
- Protective muscle spasm (muscle barriers): neck, shoulder, elbow, forearm, wrist, fingers/hand
- Myofascial test: Myofascial Mapping, fascial glide

TREATMENT

1. Muscle Energy and 'Beyond' Technique: bilateral upper extremity joints
2. Eliminate protective muscle spasm with Strain and Counterstrain:
    - Anterior thoracic (anterior T1 to T4)
    - Anterior cervicals (especially anterior C5: hold for De-Facilitated Fascial Release)
    - Lateral cervicals (especially lateral C5: hold for De-Facilitated Fascial Release)
    - Posterior cervicals
    - Elevated first rib
    - Depressed second rib (pectoralis minor)
    - Depressed third rib
    - Latissimus dorsi
    - Subscapularis
    - Anterior and posterior acromioclavicular joints
    - Supraspinatus
    - Infraspinatus
    - Biceps
3. Myofascial Release:
    - Soft Tissue Myofascial Release: transverse diaphragms (especially thoracic Inlet)
    - Soft Tissue Myofascial Release: clavipectoral release
    - Soft Tissue Myofascial Release: lateral neck hold
    - Hyoid release (4 phases)
    - Articular Fascial Release: glenohumeral joint
    - Articular Fascial Release: scapulothoracic joint
4. Tendon Release Therapy: bilateral upper extremity joints (hold for De-Facilitated Fascial Release)
5. Ligament Fiber Therapy for bilateral upper extremity joints
6. Strengthening program: especially upper quadrant
7. Posture retraining: especially focus on forward head and neck posture and protracted shoulders
8. Work hardening

COMMENTS

1. A McKenzie Program may be used to stabilize the cervical disc.
2. Occasionally, treatment of biomechanics for the pelvis and sacrum (Muscle Energy and 'Beyond' Technique) is essential to maintain cervical disc reduction.

Rotator Cuff Syndrome

ASSESSMENT

- Posture: sagittal, coronal, transverse planes: total body, focus upper quadrant
- Neurologic: focus upper quadrant
- Ranges of physiologic motions: upper quadrant, all upper quadrant joints
- Mobility testing of accessory movements: all upper quadrant joints
- Ligamentous integrity
- Apprehension/grinding tests
- Manual muscle testing
- Protective muscle spasm (muscle barriers): neck, shoulder, elbow, forearm, wrist, fingers/hand
- Myofascial test: Myofascial Mapping, fascial glide

TREATMENT

1. Muscle Energy and 'Beyond' Technique: bilateral upper extremity joints
2. Eliminate protective muscle spasm with Strain and Counterstrain:
    - Anterior thoracic (anterior T1 to T4)
    - Anterior cervicals (especially anterior C5: hold for De-Facilitated Fascial Release)
    - Lateral cervicals (especially lateral C5: hold for De-Facilitated Fascial Release)
    - Posterior cervical
    - Elevated first rib
    - Depressed second rib (pectoralis minor)
    - Depressed third rib
    - Latissimus dorsi
    - Subscapularis
    - Anterior and posterior acromioclavicular joints
    - Supraspinatus
    - Infraspinatus
    - Biceps
3. Myofascial Release:
    - Soft Tissue Myofascial Release: transverse diaphragms (especially thoracic inlet)
    - Soft Tissue Myofascial Release: clavipectoral release
    - Soft Tissue Myofascial Release: lateral neck hold
    - Hyoid release (4 phases)
    - Articular Fascial Release: glenohumeral joint
    - Articular Fascial Release: scapulothoracic joint
    - Tendon releases of rotator cuff tendons
    - Capsular release of glenohumeral joint capsule
4. Tendon Release Therapy: bilateral upper extremity joints (hold for De-Facilitated Fascial Release)
5. Ligament Fiber Therapy for bilateral upper extremity joints
6. Strengthening program: especially upper quadrant
7. Posture retraining: especially focus on forward head and neck posture and protracted shoulders
8. Stabilization of upper quadrant

Bicipital Tendinitis

ASSESSMENT

- Posture: sagittal, coronal, transverse planes: total body, focus upper quadrant
- Neurologic: focus upper quadrant
- Ranges of physiologic motions: upper quadrant, all upper quadrant joints
- Mobility testing of accessory movements: all upper quadrant joints
- Ligamentous integrity
- Apprehension/grinding tests
- Manual muscle testing
- Protective muscle spasm (muscle barriers): neck, shoulder, elbow, forearm, wrist, fingers/hand
- Myofascial test: Myofascial Mapping, fascial glide

TREATMENT

1. Muscle Energy and 'Beyond' Technique: bilateral upper extremity joints
2. Eliminate protective muscle spasm with Strain and Counterstrain:
    - Anterior thoracic (anterior T1 to T4)
    - Anterior cervicals (especially anterior C5: hold for De-Facilitated Fascial Release)
    - Lateral cervicals (especially lateral C5: hold for De-Facilitated Fascial Release)
    - Posterior cervicals
    - Elevated first rib
    - Depressed second rib (pectoralis minor)
    - Depressed third rib
    - Latissimus dorsi
    - Subscapularis
    - Anterior and posterior acromioclavicular joints
    - Supraspinatus
    - Infraspinatus
    - Biceps
    - Radial head
    - Medial epicondyle
3. Myofascial Release:
    - Soft Tissue Myofascial Release: transverse diaphragms (especially thoracic inlet)
    - Soft Tissue Myofascial Release: clavipectoral release
    - Soft Tissue Myofascial Release: lateral neck hold
    - Soft Tissue Myofascial Release: biceps
    - Soft Tissue Myofascial Release: elbow
    - Hyoid release (4 phases)
    - Articular Fascial Release: glenohumeral joint
    - Articular Fascial Release: scapulothoracic joint
    - Muscle Belly Technique: biceps
    - Tendon Release of long head of biceps
4. Tendon Release Therapy: bilateral upper extremity joints (hold for De-Facilitated Fascial Release)
5. Ligament Fiber Therapy for bilateral upper extremity joints
6. Strengthening program: especially upper quadrant
7. Posture retraining: especially focus on forward head and neck posture and protracted shoulders

Supraspinatus Tendinitis Calcification

ASSESSMENT

- Posture: sagittal, coronal, transverse planes: total body, focus upper quadrant
- Neurologic: focus upper quadrant
- Ranges of physiologic motions: upper quadrant, all upper quadrant joints
- Mobility testing of accessory movements: all upper quadrant joints
- Ligamentous integrity
- Apprehension/grinding tests
- Manual muscle testing
- Protective muscle spasm (muscle barriers): neck, shoulder, elbow, forearm, wrist, fingers/hand
- Myofascial test: Myofascial Mapping, fascial glide

TREATMENT

1. Muscle Energy and 'Beyond' Technique: bilateral upper extremity joints
2. Eliminate protective muscle spasm with Strain and Counterstrain:
    - Anterior thoracic (anterior T1 to T4)
    - Anterior cervicals (especially anterior C5: hold for De-Facilitated Fascial Release)
    - Lateral cervicals (especially lateral C5: hold for De-Facilitated Fascial Release)
    - Posterior cervicals
    - Elevated first rib
    - Depressed second rib (pectoralis minor)
    - Depressed third rib
    - Latissimus dorsi
    - Subscapularis
    - Anterior and posterior acromioclavicular joints
    - Supraspinatus
    - Infraspinatus
    - Biceps
3. Myofascial Release:
    - Soft Tissue Myofascial Release: transverse diaphragms (especially thoracic inlet)
    - Soft Tissue Myofascial Release: clavipectoral release
    - Soft Tissue Myofascial Release: lateral neck hold
    - Hyoid release (4 phases)
    - Articular Fascial Release: glenohumeral joint
    - Articular Fascial Release: scapulothoracic joint
    - Tendon release of supraspinatus tendon
4. Tendon Release Therapy: bilateral upper extremity joints (hold for De-Facilitated Fascial Release)
5. Ligament Fiber Therapy for bilateral upper extremity joints
6. Iontophoresis: acetic acid (positive electrode on supraspinatus tendon)
7. Strengthening program: especially upper quadrant
8. Posture retraining: especially focus on forward head and neck posture and protracted shoulders

Dysphagia

ASSESSMENT

- Posture: sagittal, coronal, transverse planes: total body, focus upper quadrant
- Neurologic: focus upper quadrant
- Ranges of physiologic motions: upper quadrant, all upper quadrant joints
- Mobility testing of accessory movements: all upper quadrant joints
- Ligamentous integrity
- Apprehension/grinding tests
- Manual muscle testing
- Protective muscle spasm (muscle barriers): neck, shoulder, elbow, forearm, wrist, fingers/hand
- Myofascial test: Myofascial Mapping, fascial glide

TREATMENT

1. Muscle Energy and 'Beyond' Technique: bilateral upper extremity joints
2. Eliminate protective muscle spasm with Strain and Counterstrain:
    - Anterior thoracic (anterior T1 to T4)
    - Anterior cervicals (especially anterior C5: hold for De-Facilitated Fascial Release)
    - Lateral cervicals (especially lateral C5: hold for De-Facilitated Fascial Release)
    - Posterior cervicals
    - Elevated first rib
    - Depressed second rib (pectoralis minor)
    - Depressed third rib
    - Latissimus dorsi
    - Subscapularis
    - Anterior and posterior acromioclavicular joints
    - Supraspinatus
    - Infraspinatus
    - Biceps
    - Do every anterior cervical technique and perform a De-Facilitated Fascial Release for each
3. Myofascial Release:
    - Soft Tissue Myofascial Release: transverse diaphragms (especially thoracic inlet)
    - Soft Tissue Myofascial Release: clavipectoral release
    - Soft Tissue Myofascial Release: lateral neck hold
    - Hyoid release (4 phases)
4. Tendon Release Therapy: bilateral upper extremity joints (hold for De-Facilitated Fascial Release)
5. Ligament Fiber Therapy for bilateral upper extremity joints
6. Myofunctional therapy for strengthening, proprioception, exteroception, and coordination of the hyoid system (References: Dan Garliner, *Myofunctional Therapy;* Rocabado, *"Six by Six" Protocol*)
7. Strengthening Program: especially upper quadrant
8. Posture retraining: especially focus on forward head and neck posture and protracted shoulders

Protracted Shoulder Girdle

ASSESSMENT

- Posture: sagittal, coronal, transverse planes: total body, focus upper quadrant
- Neurologic: focus upper quadrant
- Ranges of physiologic motions: all upper quadrant joints
- Mobility testing of accessory movements: all upper quadrant joints
- Ligamentous integrity
- Apprehension/grinding tests
- Manual muscle testing
- Protective muscle spasm (muscle barriers): neck, shoulder, elbow, forearm, wrist, fingers/hand
- Myofascial test: Myofascial Mapping, fascial glide

TREATMENT

1. Muscle Energy and 'Beyond' Technique: bilateral upper extremity joints
2. Eliminate protective muscle spasm with Strain and Counterstrain:
    - Anterior thoracic (anterior T1 to T4)
    - Anterior cervicals (especially anterior C5: hold for De-Facilitated Fascial Release)
    - Lateral cervicals (especially lateral C5: hold for De-Facilitated Fascial Release)
    - Posterior cervicals
    - Elevated first rib
    - Depressed second rib (pectoralis minor)
    - Depressed third rib
    - Latissimus dorsi
    - Subscapularis
    - Anterior and posterior acromioclavicular joints
    - Supraspinatus
    - Infraspinatus
    - Biceps
3. Myofascial Release:
    - Soft Tissue Myofascial Release: transverse diaphragms (especially thoracic inlet)
    - Soft Tissue Myofascial Release: clavipectoral release
    - Soft Tissue Myofascial Release: lateral neck hold
    - Hyoid release (4 phases)
    - Articular Fascial Release: glenohumeral joint
    - Articular Fascial Release: scapulothoracic joint
4. Tendon Release Therapy: bilateral upper extremity joints (hold for De-Facilitated Fascial Release)
5. Ligament Fiber Therapy for bilateral upper extremity joints
6. Strengthening program: especially upper quadrant
7. Posture retraining: especially focus on forward head and neck posture and protracted shoulders

Tennis Elbow

ASSESSMENT

- Posture: sagittal, coronal, transverse planes: total body, focus upper quadrant
- Neurologic: focus upper quadrant
- Ranges of physiologic motions: all upper quadrant joints
- Mobility testing of accessory movements: all upper quadrant joints
- Ligamentous integrity
- Apprehension/grinding tests
- Manual muscle testing
- Protective muscle spasm (muscle barriers): neck, shoulder, elbow, forearm, wrist, fingers/hand
- Myofascial test: Myofascial Mapping, fascial glide

TREATMENT

1. Muscle Energy and 'Beyond' Technique: bilateral upper extremity joints
2. Eliminate protective muscle spasm with Strain and Counterstrain:
    - Anterior thoracic (anterior T1 to T4)
    - Anterior cervicals (especially anterior C5: hold for De-Facilitated Fascial Release)
    - Lateral cervicals (especially Lateral C5: hold for De-Facilitated Fascial Release)
    - Posterior cervicals
    - Elevated first rib
    - Depressed second rib (pectoralis minor)
    - Depressed third rib
    - Latissimus dorsi
    - Subscapularis
    - Anterior and posterior acromioclavicular joints
    - Supraspinatus
    - Infraspinatus
    - Biceps
    - Radial head
    - Anterior carpals
3. Myofascial Release:
    - Soft Tissue Myofascial Release: transverse diaphragms (especially thoracic inlet)
    - Soft Tissue Myofascial Release: clavipectoral release
    - Soft Tissue Myofascial Release: lateral neck hold
    - Soft Tissue Myofascial Release: elbow
    - Soft Tissue Myofascial Release: anterior compartment
    - Soft Tissue Myofascial Release: carpal tunnel
    - Hyoid release (4 phases)
    - Articular Fascial Release: glenohumeral joint
    - Articular Fascial Release: scapulothoracic joint
    - Articular Fascial Release: all elbow joints
    - Articular Fascial Release: wrist joint
    - Muscle Belly Technique: biceps and triceps together
    - Muscle Belly Technique: brachioradialis
    - Tendon Release: brachioradiolis tendon
    - Ligament Release: lateral ligaments of elbow joint
    - Radioulnar Hanging Technique
4. Tendon Release Therapy: bilateral upper extremity joints (hold for De-Facilitated Fascial Release)
5. Ligament Fiber Therapy for bilateral upper extremity joints
6. Iontophoresis: Iodex: iodine methyl salicylate (negative electrode) and acetic acid (positive electrode) to brachioradialis tendon
7. Strengthening program: especially upper quadrant
8. Posture retraining: especially focus on forward head and neck posture and protracted shoulders

Golfer's Elbow

ASSESSMENT

- Posture: sagittal, coronal, transverse planes: total body, focus upper quadrant
- Neurologic: focus upper quadrant
- Ranges of physiologic motions: all upper quadrant joints
- Mobility testing of accessory movements: all upper quadrant joints
- Ligamentous integrity
- Apprehension/grinding tests
- Manual muscle testing
- Protective muscle spasm (muscle barriers): neck, shoulder, elbow, forearm, wrist, fingers/hand
- Myofascial test: Myofascial Mapping, fascial glide

TREATMENT

1. Muscle Energy and 'Beyond' Technique: bilateral upper extremity joints
2. Eliminate protective muscle spasm with Strain and Counterstrain:
    - Anterior thoracic (anterior T1 to T4)
    - Anterior cervicals (especially anterior C5: hold for De-Facilitated Fascial Release)
    - Lateral cervicals (especially lateral C5: hold for De-Facilitated Fascial Release)
    - Posterior cervicals
    - Elevated first rib
    - Depressed second rib (pectoralis minor)
    - Depressed third rib
    - Latissimus dorsi
    - Subscapularis
    - Anterior and posterior acromioclavicular joints
    - Supraspinatus
    - Infraspinatus
    - Biceps
    - Radial head
    - Medial epicondyle
    - Anterior carpals
3. Myofascial Release:
    - Soft Tissue Myofascial Release: transverse diaphragms (especially thoracic inlet)
    - Soft Tissue Myofascial Release: clavipectoral release
    - Soft Tissue Myofascial Release: lateral neck hold
    - Soft Tissue Myofascial Release: elbow
    - Soft Tissue Myofascial Release: anterior compartment
    - Soft Tissue Myofascial Release: carpal tunnel
    - Hyoid release (4 phases)
    - Articular Fascial Release: glenohumeral joint
    - Articular Fascial Release: scapulothoracic joint
    - Articular Fascial Release: all elbow joints
    - Articular Fascial Release: wrist joint
    - Muscle Belly Technique: biceps and triceps together
    - Ligament Release: lateral ligaments of elbow joint
    - Radioulnar Hanging Technique
4. Tendon Release Therapy: bilateral upper extremity joints (hold for De-Facilitated Fascial Release)
5. Ligament Fiber Therapy for bilateral upper extremity joints
6. Strengthening program: especially upper quadrant
7. Posture retraining: especially focus on forward head and neck posture and protracted shoulders

Anterior Compartment Syndrome

ASSESSMENT

- Posture: sagittal, coronal, transverse planes: total body, focus upper quadrant
- Neurologic: focus upper quadrant
- Ranges of physiologic motions: all upper quadrant joints
- Mobility testing of accessory movements: all upper quadrant joints
- Ligamentous integrity
- Apprehension/grinding tests
- Manual muscle testing
- Protective muscle spasm (muscle barriers): neck, shoulder, elbow, forearm, wrist, fingers/hand
- Myofascial test: Myofascial Mapping, fascial glide

TREATMENT

1. Muscle Energy and 'Beyond' Technique: bilateral upper extremity joints
2. Eliminate protective muscle spasm with Strain and Counterstrain:
    - Anterior thoracic (anterior T1 to T4)
    - Anterior cervicals (especially anterior C5: hold for De-Facilitated Fascial Release)
    - Lateral cervicals (especially lateral C5: hold for De-Facilitated Fascial Release)
    - Posterior cervicals
    - Elevated first rib
    - Depressed second rib (pectoralis minor)
    - Depressed third rib
    - Latissimus dorsi
    - Subscapularis
    - Anterior and posterior Acromioclavicular joints
    - Supraspinatus
    - Infraspinatus
    - Biceps
    - Radial head
    - Anterior carpals
3. Myofascial Release:
    - Soft Tissue Myofascial Release: transverse diaphragms (especially thoracic inlet)
    - Soft Tissue Myofascial Release: clavipectoral release
    - Soft Tissue Myofascial Release: lateral neck hold
    - Soft Tissue Myofascial Release: elbow
    - Soft Tissue Myofascial Release: anterior compartment
    - Soft Tissue Myofascial Release: carpal tunnel
    - Hyoid release (4 phases)
    - Articular Fascial Release: glenohumeral joint
    - Articular Fascial Release: scapulothoracic joint
    - Articular Fascial Release: all elbow joints
    - Articular Fascial Release: wrist joint
    - Muscle Belly Technique: biceps and triceps together
    - Ligament Release: lateral ligaments of elbow joint
    - Radioulnar Hanging Technique
4. Tendon Release Therapy: bilateral upper extremity joints (hold for De-Facilitated Fascial Release)
5. Ligament Fiber Therapy for bilateral upper extremity joints
6. Strengthening program: especially upper quadrant
7. Posture retraining: especially focus on forward head and neck posture and protracted shoulders

Carpal Tunnel Syndrome

ASSESSMENT

- Posture: sagittal, coronal, transverse planes: total body, focus upper quadrant
- Neurologic: focus upper quadrant
- Ranges of physiologic motions: all upper quadrant joints
- Mobility testing of accessory movements: all upper quadrant joints
- Ligamentous integrity
- Apprehension/grinding tests
- Manual muscle testing
- Protective muscle spasm (muscle barriers): neck, shoulder, elbow, forearm, wrist, fingers/hand
- Myofascial test: Myofascial Mapping, fascial glide

TREATMENT

1. Muscle Energy and 'Beyond' Technique: bilateral upper extremity joints
2. Eliminate protective muscle spasm with Strain and Counterstrain:
    - Anterior thoracic (anterior T1 to T4)
    - Anterior cervicals specially anterior C5: hold for De-Facilitated Fascial Release)
    - Lateral cervicals (especially lateral C5: hold for De-Facilitated Fascial Release)
    - Posterior cervicals
    - Elevated first rib
    - Depressed second rib (pectoralis minor)
    - Depressed third rib
    - Latissimus dorsi
    - Subscapularis
    - Anterior and posterior acromioclavicular joints
    - Supraspinatus
    - Infraspinatus
    - Biceps
    - Radial head
    - Anterior carpals
    - Posterior carpals
3. Myofascial Release:
    - Soft Tissue Myofascial Release: transverse diaphragms (especially thoracic inlet)
    - Soft Tissue Myofascial Release: clavipectoral release
    - Soft Tissue Myofascial Release: lateral neck hold
    - Soft Tissue Myofascial Release: elbow
    - Soft Tissue Myofascial Release: anterior compartment
    - Soft Tissue Myofascial Release: carpal tunnel
    - Hyoid release (4 phases)
    - Articular Fascial Release: glenohumeral joint
    - Articular Fascial Release: scapulothoracic joint
    - Articular Fascial Release: all elbow joints
    - Articular Fascial Release: wrist joint
    - Tendon Release: anterior and posterior tendons crossing wrist joint
    - Retinaculum Technique
4. Tendon Release Therapy: bilateral upper extremity joints (hold for De-Facilitated Fascial Release)
5. Ligament Fiber Therapy for bilateral upper extremity joints
6. Strengthening program: especially upper quadrant
7. Posture retraining: especially focus on forward head and neck posture and protracted shoulders

De Quervain's Syndrome

ASSESSMENT

- Posture: sagittal, coronal, transverse planes: total body, focus upper quadrant
- Neurologic: focus upper quadrant
- Ranges of physiologic motions: all upper quadrant joints
- Mobility testing of accessory movements: all upper quadrant joints
- Ligamentous integrity
- Apprehension/grinding tests
- Manual muscle testing
- Protective muscle spasm (muscle barriers): neck, shoulder, elbow, forearm, wrist, fingers/hand
- Myofascial test: Myofascial Mapping, fascial glide

TREATMENT

1. Muscle Energy and 'Beyond' Technique: bilateral upper extremity joints
2. Eliminate protective muscle spasm with Strain and Counterstrain:
    - Anterior thoracic (anterior T1 to T4)
    - Anterior cervicals (especially anterior C5: hold for De-Facilitated Fascial Release)
    - Lateral cervicals (especially lateral C5: hold for De-Facilitated Fascial Release)
    - Posterior cervicals
    - Elevated first rib
    - Depressed second rib (pectoralis minor)
    - Depressed third rib
    - Latissimus dorsi
    - Subscapularis
    - Anterior and posterior acromioclavicular joints
    - Supraspinatus
    - Infraspinatus
    - Biceps
    - Radial head
    - Anterior carpals
    - Posterior carpals
    - First Carpometacarpal Technique
3. Myofascial Release:
    - Soft Tissue Myofascial Release: transverse diaphragms especially thoracic Inlet)
    - Soft Tissue Myofascial Release: clavipectoral release
    - Soft Tissue Myofascial Release: lateral neck hold
    - Soft Tissue Myofascial Release: elbow
    - Soft Tissue Myofascial Release: anterior compartment
    - Soft Tissue Myofascial Release: carpal tunnel
    - Hyoid release (4 phases)
    - Articular Fascial Release: glenohumeral joint
    - Articular Fascial Release: scapulothoracic joint
    - Articular Fascial Release: all elbow joints
    - Articular Fascial Release: wrist joint
    - Articular Fascial Release: first carpometacarpal joint
    - Tendon Release: abductor and adductor thumb tendons
4. Tendon Release Therapy: bilateral upper extremity joints (hold for De-Facilitated Fascial Release)
5. Ligament Fiber Therapy for bilateral upper extremity joints
6. Strengthening program: especially upper quadrant
7. Posture retraining: especially focus on forward head and neck posture and protracted shoulders
8. Hand functional therapy

Spasticity of the Upper Extremity

ASSESSMENT

- Posture: sagittal, coronal, transverse planes: total body, focus upper quadrant
- Neurologic: focus upper quadrant, focus on spastic synergic pattern which includes: flexed cervical spine; elevated and protracted shoulder girdle; flexed, adducted, and internally rotated shoulder joint (assess for anterior and caudal subluxed hemiplegic shoulder; flexed elbow; pronated forearm; flexed and ulnar deviated wrist; flexed and adducted thumb; flexed fingers)
- Ranges of physiologic motions: all upper quadrant joints
- Mobility testing of accessory movements: all upper quadrant joints
- Ligamentous integrity
- Apprehension/grinding tests
- Manual muscle testing
- Hypertonicity: cervical flexors, supraspinatus, pectoralis minor, latissimus dorsi; subscapularis, biceps, and all flexors
- Myofascial test: Myofascial Mapping, fascial glide

TREATMENT

1. Muscle Energy and 'Beyond' Technique: bilateral upper extremity joints
2. Eliminate Protective Muscle Spasm with Strain and Counterstrain:
    - Anterior thoracic (anterior T1 to T4)
    - Anterior cervicals (especially anterior C5: hold for De-Facilitated Fascial Release)
    - Lateral cervicals (especially lateral C5: hold for De-Facilitated Fascial Release)
    - Posterior cervicals
    - Elevated first rib
    - Depressed second rib (pectoralis minor)
    - Depressed third rib
    - Latissimus dorsi
    - Subscapularis
    - Anterior and posterior acromioclavicular joints
    - Supraspinatus
    - Infraspinatus
    - Interosseous muscles
3. Myofascial Release:
    - Soft Tissue Myofascial Release: transverse diaphragms (especially thoracic inlet)
    - Soft Tissue Myofascial Release: clavipectoral release
    - Soft Tissue Myofascial Release: lateral neck hold
    - Soft Tissue Myofascial Release: all upper extremity joints
    - Hyoid release (4 phases)
    - Articular Fascial Release: all upper extremity joints
    - Articular Fascial Release: scapulothoracic joint
4. Tendon Release Therapy: bilateral upper extremity joints (hold for De-Facilitated Fascial Release)
5. Ligament Fiber Therapy for bilateral upper extremity joints
6. Strengthening Program: especially upper quadrant
7. Posture retraining: especially focus on forward head and neck posture and protracted shoulders
8. Hand functional therapy

INDEX

Q

R

S

T

U

V

W

DIALOGUES IN CONTEMPORARY REHABILITATION

History of Dialogues in Contemporary Rehabilitation

DCR is the company for Integrative Manual Therapy, the Integrated Systems Approach, Integrative Diagnostics, and Functional and Structural Rehabilitation. Founded in the early 1980s by Mary Fiorentino, O.T.,R. Sharon (Weiselfish) Giammatteo initiated a transformation in the educational process incorporated by DCR in 1986, when she received ownership from Mary. Faculty of DCR are trained in all areas of manual therapy; they are experts in the fields of orthopedics and sports medicine, chronic pain, neuro-rehabilitation, pediatrics, geriatrics, women's and men's health issues, cardiopulmonary rehabilitation and more. Almost 100 percent of the material offered by DCR has been developed, research and present-day results performed, at Regional Physical Therapy in Connecticut.

DCR Mission Statement

DCR offers hope, practice and purpose. Our goal is recovery; our intention is learning, teaching, and understanding. Our field of accomplishment is extended to client, family, community and world. We accept tomorrow's knowledge as today's quest. We are not hindered by greed, inhibitions, or belief systems. We are multi-denominational, cross-cultural, and non-racial in orientation. We wish to facilitate recovery from dysfunction through growth and development.

DCR Seminars

Biomechanics with: Muscle Energy and 'Beyond' Technique

MET1: Pelvis, Sacrum and Spine

MET2: Upper and Lower Extremities and Rib Cage

MET3: Advanced Biomechanics: Sacrum and Spine

MET4: Type III Biomechanical Dysfunction: Spine and Extremities and Bone Bruises

Muscle and Circulation with Strain and Counterstrain Technique

SCS1: Strain and Counterstrain for Orthopedics and Neurologic Patient

SCS2: Advanced Strain and Counterstrain for Autonomic Nervous System

Connective Tissue with Myofascial Release, The 3-Planar Fascial Fulcrum Technique

MFR1: Myofascial Release for Orthopedic, Neurologic, Geriatric Patient

MFR2: Myofascial Mapping for Integrative Diagnostics

Peripheral Nerve Tissue Tension: Hypomobility and Fibrosis

NTT2: Neural Tissue Tension Technique

Cranial and the Craniosacral System with: The Cranial Therapy Series

CTS1: Osseous, Suture, Joint and Membrane

CTS2: Membrane, Fluid, Facial Vault and Cranial Gear-Complex

CTS3: Cranial Diaphragm Compression Syndromes; CSF Fluid: Production, Distribution and Absorption; Immunology

CTS4: Neuronal Regeneration, Cranial Nerves, and Neurotransmission

CTSA1: Postural Reflexes

CTSA2: Vasculature in the Brain

CTSA3: The Eye

Organs with Visceral Mobilization

VMET1: Visceral Mobilization with Muscle Energy and 'Beyond'—Focus GI Tract

VMET2: Women's and Men's Health Issues

VMET3: Respiratory Rehabilitation

VMET4: Cardiac Habilitation

VMET5: The Liver

The Lymphatic System

LYM1: Congestion Therapy

LYM2: Immune Preference

Compression Syndromes

COMP1: Compression Syndromes of the Upper Extremities

COMP2: Compression Syndromes of the Lower Extremities

COMP3: Diaphragm Compression Syndromes

Neuro-Rehabilitation

DMT: Developmental Manual Therapy for the Neurologic Patient

Integrative Diagnostics

IDS: Integrative Diagnostic Series: Myofascial Mapping, Neurofascial Process, Rx Plans

IDAP: Integrative Diagnostics for Applied Psychosynthesis

IDLB: Integrative Diagnostics for Lower Back

Integrative Seminars

IMTS: Integrative Manual Therapy for Neck, Thoracic Outlet, Shoulder and Upper Extremity

IMTUE/LESM: Integrative Manual Therapy for Upper and Lower Extremities in Sports Medicine

IMTCCC: Integrative Manual Therapy for Craniocervical, Craniofacial, Craniomandibular

Functional Rehabilitation

Therapeutic Horizons: The Brain (BANM); The Heart (BACM); The Pelvis (BANRA); Advanced Levels 1–3 (BAAL1–3)

NES & DCR Offer Adjunct Educational Material in Integrative Manual Therapy

Books

Manual Therapy for the Pelvis, Sacrum, Cervical, Thoracic and Lumbar Spine, with Muscle Energy Technique—A Contemporary Clinical Analysis of Biomechanics by Sharon Weiselfish, Ph.D., P.T.

Integrative Manual Therapy for the Autonomic Nervous System and Related Disorders by Thomas Giammatteo, D.C. P.T., and Sharon (Weiselfish) Giammatteo, Ph.D., P.T.

Integrative Manual Therapy for the Upper and Lower Extremities, Introducing Synergic Pattern Release with Strain and Counterstrain Technique and Muscle Energy and 'Beyond' Technique for the Peripheral Joints by Sharon (Weiselfish) Giammatteo, Ph.D., P.T., edited by Thomas Giammatteo, D.C., P.T.

Videos

By Sharon (Weiselfish) Giammatteo, Ph.D., P.T.
Produced by Northeast Seminars

Muscle Energy Technique Series

#1 Pelvis

#2 Sacrum

#3 Thoracic and Lumbar Spine

#4 Cervical and Thoracic Spine

#5 Strain and Counterstrain for the Orthopedic and Neurologic Patient

#6 Myofascial Release, the 3-Planar Fascial Fulcrum Approach, for the Orthopedic, Neurologic and Geriatric Patient

#7 Advanced Manual Therapy for the Low Back

#8 Integrative Manual Therapy: A Patient in Process

#9 Manual Therapy for the Low Back: Standards for the Health Care Industry for the 21st Century

#10 Muscle Energy and 'Beyond' Technique for the Upper Extremities

#11 Muscle Energy and 'Beyond' Technique for the Lower Extremities

For further information regarding educational videos, please contact Northeast Seminars at:

Northeast Seminars
P.O. Box 522
East Hampstead, NH 03826
Tel: 800-272-2044 / Fax: 603-329-7045
E-mail: neseminar@aol.com
Website: www.neseminars.com

For further information regarding DCR products and seminars, please contact DCR at:

DCR
Dialogues in Contemporary Rehabilitation
800 Cottage Grove Road, Suite 211
Bloomfield, CT 06002
Tel: 860-243-5220 / Fax: 860-243-5304
E-mail: dcrhealth@aol.com
Website: www.dcrhealth.com